Mindfulness

and Care of the Dying

Mindfulness
and Care of the Dying

Dr. Tan Seng Beng

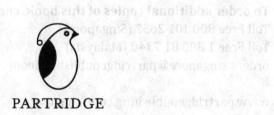

PARTRIDGE

To order additional copies of this book, contact
Toll Free 800 101 2657 (Singapore)
Toll Free 1 800 81 7340 (Malaysia)
orders.singapore@partridgepublishing.com

www.partridgepublishing.com/singapore

Be like a sunflower

And bring joy to the world

CONTENTS

CONTENTS

Foreword

Yong Chen Joyce

I was asked a peculiar question by Seng Beng on the first day of my attachment with the palliative care team. "How would you like to die?" All I could think of was, anything but cancer.

My mother was diagnosed with leukemia in July 2014. She fought the cancer with every ounce of energy she had and soldiered on. Due to her weakened immune system, she had to stay in an isolation room alone for three months while receiving treatment for her cancer. It was truly a challenging time for her but she never once backed down. Six months on, we were told the wonderful news that her cancer was cured. We were overjoyed. All our efforts paid off. Our family was finally complete again.

My mother was an incredible woman. She was one of the kindest souls that I have known. I never saw her say no to anyone in need of a helping hand. She was always a beacon of light bringing hope into the lives of the people she touched. She taught her children to be fearless and she always pushed us to reach for our dreams. She celebrated both our triumphs and failures; and constantly reminded us that we were loved no matter what.

There are some moments in life when you know that things will never be the same again. This was one of those moments. Shortly after my mother was cured of her leukemia, she was diagnosed with terminal lung cancer. We were told that it was likely caused by one of the drugs used during the treatment of her leukemia. Her survival rate would be measured in months, not years.

I was furious that medicine had failed my mother. It was ironic that the very same treatment that gave my mother life, was taking it away. We were absolutely devastated. Heartbroken, we searched for a second opinion. Then, a third and a fourth opinion, which all came back with the same verdict. This couldn't be happening. What were the odds? How could anyone get two different cancers in less than a year?

The 'C' word, again. This cancer was different. There was no hope for a cure this time around. There was no hope. The cycles of chemotherapy were endless. First line of treatment failed. Second line failed. Third line failed as well. All we kept hearing month after month was "Your cancer has progressed. This treatment no longer works." It seemed like wherever we turned, it was a dead end. We had no choice but to come face to face with the unpredictability and fragility of my mother's life.

When a loved one was given a time limit on how long she could live, you started living life with a sense of urgency. Our entire family did. We dropped everything on hand to be with my mother. We had some good days, some bad and some just downright horrible.

It was during this emotionally trying time that I was introduced to mindfulness by Seng Beng and his palliative care team. I joined the palliative care team hoping to better prepare myself for my mother's impending death. As a medical student, I have witnessed many deaths in the hospital but none of the experiences prepared me for my own mother's death.

The day my mother stopped eating, I broke down. Anything that went into her mouth, came right back out. Was it really happening? Was she dying? This was just too soon. This couldn't be happening. I couldn't bear the thought of losing her. The air was knocked out of my lungs and I felt like I couldn't breathe.

It was then that I recalled an exercise I was taught during the palliative care attachment: Always be aware of your breath. Whenever you find yourself lost in the thoughts of your past, where you cannot change; or future, which you have no control, you just need to remember to breathe. Live your life one breath at a time, moment by moment. You just need to breathe.

When I focused on my breathing, time flowed a little slower. I felt like I have more time and space to comprehend the events that were happening around me. Mindfulness gave me a sense of serenity in the chaos that I felt. There was something inherently powerful in death that drew me to contemplate the meaning and purpose of my existence. Mindfulness provided me with a safe space for quiet reflection and better insight. It was between these breaths that I was able to fully experience the wonder and beauty that blossomed towards the end of my mother's life.

On July 2016, my mother was admitted for a minor surgery to help relieve her breathlessness. Little did I know that when I said goodbye that night, it would be the last time I could ever speak to her again. We couldn't wake her up the next day. My mother breathed her last breath with all her loved ones surrounding her. She passed away days before her 55th birthday.

"The death of a mother is the first sorrow wept without her."

The only comfort I had was that there were no words left unsaid between us. When you lose your loved ones, you never really lose certain memories or certain parts of their personality. To this day, I still remember the way she smiles, her off-pitched singing and dorky dance moves. I think the death of a mother is not something you can really get over. You just learn to understand what it means. I learnt to live and love better. I am blessed to have known and loved this woman that gave me life. I will always keep the times and memories we have close to my heart.

My mother's death was a transformative experience that was simultaneously heart-breaking yet profound. I have truly experienced a beautiful end to my mother's life. My hope is that, through this book, Mindfulness and Care of the Dying, you too will be able to find the beauty in life, in all situations, including death.

Preface

Death is an illusion. We think it is real, but it is not. Our bodies are made of organic compounds. Organic compounds are made of elements. Elements are made of particles. Particles are made of subatomic particles, such as quarks and leptons – the subatomic particles of matter. And subatomic particles are made of vibration of energy. Likewise, our minds are made of thoughts and feelings. Thoughts and feelings are made of neuronal activities. Neuronal activities are electrical activities. Electrical activities are electromagnetic waves. Electromagnetic waves are carried by photons – one of the subatomic particles of force, belongs to the gauge bosons group. Photons are also vibration of energy. We are all vibration of energy in different frequencies. Death is unreal.

Death is a drop of take-away Starbucks coffee spilled on the floor when we rush to work. It often evaporates slowly, leaving a light brown stain with a dark rim. The rim can be spiky, like the envelope of a virus. The thing is, no one really cares about this drop. Some even step on it, unintentionally. Some mop it off so no one can see it. Death is a flash of lightning in the sky that catches our eyes when we are stuck in a traffic jam. When we are strong and healthy, we never think of death. But death can strike us like a lightning when we are most unprepared.

Death is a bubble blown from our all-time familiar Wrigley's Doublemint bubble gum. We all enjoy chewing it, but it is not so easy to blow it. First, we need to roll the gum into a ball with our tongue. Second, we need to push our tongue through it. Third, we need to blow air into it. The thing is, we can't stop blowing once it expands. And we won't be able to know the exact time it will pop all over our face.

Death is a joke. Even though it is an illusion, we cling to it as real. Even though it is a display of energy vibrations, like a show, like dream, like the firecrackers, but we never enjoy it. Not only we never enjoy it, we try to avoid it at all costs, to the extent of giving pressures to the doctors to keep us alive, or blaming the doctors if they can't. We create a lot of electrical activities of suffering for ourselves and for others around us. The nature of our mind is inherently free from stress and suffering. They are merely vibrations of high frequency energy. We are brilliantly sane, from the fundamental point of view. But the slight twist in our thinking process creates this whole illimitable display of neuronal activities of suffering during death and dying.

How can we come out of this trap of suffering caused by death and dying? Mindfulness is one way. Our conscious capacity to regulate or cease the electrical activities of suffering gives us opportunity to escape this trap. Based on the original text on mindfulness – the *Satipatthana Sutta*, the first half of the book is written to guide us in increasing our capacity to regulate our own neurological activities for our own good, in a step-by-step manner. The second half of the book is written to allow us to improve the capacity further while we are caring for others, particularly the dying. My wish for the book is to help people cultivate mindfulness in their life and their works of caring. May the book help to reduce the electrical activities of suffering of ourselves and others, and bring joy and happiness to the world, like sunflowers!

May you be happy and at ease,

Dr Tan Seng Beng

8th March 2018

Mindfulness

Introduction

Before we start to discuss mindfulness-based supportive therapy (MBST), first we have to develop a thorough understanding of what is meant by mindfulness – the theory of mindfulness. Second we have to spend a lot of time to familiarize ourselves with the experience of mindfulness – the practice of mindfulness. Third and most importantly, we ourselves have to live mindfully – the embodiment of mindfulness in our day-to-day life. If we live unconsciously in a busily and forgetful manner, it is difficult to practice mindfulness-based supportive therapy at work. So, to start with, we need to build a strong foundation of mindfulness for ourselves, and this can be achieved by reading, practicing and living the first half of this book.

Ice-cream and mindfulness

If we read a lot about mindfulness but never really practice it, we are like knowing what ice-cream is but never really taste it. If we practice mindfulness during formal sitting sessions but never really live our life mindfully, we are like tasting vanilla ice-cream but never really try all the other flavors of Häagen-Dazs.

Mindfulness is the translation of the Pali word '*sati*', which means attention. Attention is a natural ability of our mind. When we see a flower, if we pay full attention to the flower, then, we are being mindful of the presence of this wonderful flower. But how is this attention different from our day-to-day attention. *Sati* is a form of introspective attention. That means the direction of the attention is inward, looking inside the workings of our mind in order to free ourselves from all negative mental states, but not to abuse our attention capacity to achieve selfish goals.

Sati also means to remember, to remember to come back to the present moment, to be present for what life is, in the here and now. We spend a significant amount of time, if not all the time, thinking about something, about the past or about the future. In mindfulness, we remember to come back to our senses and to live in the present moment, in the here and now. But it does not mean we cannot think about the past or the future. It simply means we are fully aware of what we are doing or thinking right now. When we are thinking about the past we know we are thinking about the past right now; or when we are dreaming about the future we are fully aware we are dreaming about the future.

Mindfulness has been shown to reduce stress in a variety of conditions. It helps us to improve pain acceptance, tiredness, sleep problems, sadness and worry. It also helps us to be more present for every moment of our life. It makes us feel more alive. And it reveals to us the inner world of our mind so we can make full use of it to achieve a long-lasting kind of happiness or well-being. These are some of the benefits of practicing mindfulness.

The original text on the teachings of mindfulness is called *Satipatthana Sutta*. *Satipatthana* means mindfulness that is firmly established. It is a form of attention that sinks deep into the object of attention like a rock sinking into the bottom of water instead of just floating on the surface of the object like a ball wobbling on the surface of water. When we practice mindfulness, we try to establish it firmly on the object of our choice and also the object that becomes prominent at the present moment.

The *Satipatthana Sutta* describes four foundations or fields of practice to establish mindfulness in a systematic manner:

- Mindfulness of the body (*kayanupassana*)
- Mindfulness of feelings (*vedananupassana*)
- Mindfulness of mind (*cittanupassana*)
- Mindfulness of thoughts (*dhammanupassana*)

M&M's chocolate and mindfulness

Although people said everything in the universe is made of atoms, mindfulness is not. Mindfulness is made of mini-mindfulness moments (mmms). It is a little bit like the M&M's chocolate, mmm, so delicious. We should start practicing mindfulness with these tiny moments of mindfulness, these tiny moments of mmms. Every time we remember, we come back to the present moment. Every time we are aware, we come back to these mmms.

The goals of practicing mindfulness

The *satipatthana* is a systematic way in the training of attention. It is the direct path for the purification of the mind, for the overcoming of sorrow and lamentation, for the relief of physical and mental suffering, for seeing things as they are, and for the experiencing of the complete cessation of stress. These are the five goals of practicing mindfulness. If we practice mindfulness to achieve a selfish reason or to harm others, we are not practicing right mindfulness (*samma sati*), but wrong mindfulness (*miccha sati*). It is like mindfully lying to our friend or robbing a bank. The underlying motivation in practicing mindfulness is crucial. We have to practice mindfulness with a wholesome motivation.

What are the four foundations of mindfulness?

Satipatthana Sutta: In regard to the body, one abides observing the body as the body, ardent, clearly knowing, mindful, removing greed and anger. In regard to feelings, one abides observing feelings as feelings, ardent, clearly knowing, mindful, removing greed and anger. In regard to the mind, one abides observing mind as mind, ardent, clearly knowing, mindful, removing greed and anger. In regard to thoughts, one abides observing thoughts as thoughts, ardent, clearly knowing, mindful, removing greed and anger.

When it comes to reading the instructions from the *Sutta*, it is recommended to read them slowly and mindfully. That means when we are reading we know we are reading. We are not carried away by our judgments, like thinking how come there are so many repetitions. These repetitions are systematic instructions on the practice of mindfulness. If we read them mindfully, we are already practicing mindfulness. So when we see the instructions from the *Sutta*, please slow down and read them mindfully.

The four foundations of mindfulness

First, I studied at Gopeng Kindergarten. Then, I did my primary education at Gopeng Man Ming. After that, I went to Idris Shah Secondary School for three years before I moved to Ipoh Sam Tet to further my studies. After completing my secondary education, I did medicine in University of Malaya, Kuala Lumpur. In 2000, I graduated and began my medicine career. Likewise, in practicing mindfulness, we start with mindfulness of the body, followed by mindfulness of feelings, mind and thoughts. Once we have built our four foundations, we move on to MBST.

The relationships between characters and the foundations

For those who are emotional and less intellectual, mindfulness of the body suits them best. For those who are emotional and highly intellectual, mindfulness of feelings is better for them. For those who are calm and less intellectual, mindfulness of mind is good for them. For those who are calm and highly intellectual, mindfulness of thoughts is the best.

These correlations not only can be applied to specific characters, they could be applied to current states of mind too. We can practice mindfulness of the body when we are emotional and sluggish; mindfulness of feelings when we are emotional and sharp; mindfulness of mind when we are calm and sluggish; and mindfulness of thoughts when we are calm and sharp.

The four mental qualities in establishing mindfulness

According to the definition of mindfulness, four specific mental qualities must be established in the practice of *satipatthana*, namely ardency (*atapi*), clear comprehension (*sampajanna*), mindfulness (*sati*), and the removing of greed and anger (*vineyya abhijjhadomanassa*). All four mental qualities are needed in the practice of mindfulness.

In establishing mindfulness, first we need to be ardent, diligent and make effort. *Atapi* in Pali means burning the mental defilements. *Atapi* comes from the word *atapa* which means heat. Heat here means effort. We must make effort to be mindful. Without effort, we cannot be mindful. Heat also means energy. The energy needed should be just enough to sustain the practice of mindfulness in a balanced manner, not too tensed up and not too relaxed. Just like when we are tuning our guitar strings, the music played won't be very nice if the strings are too tight or too loose. This *atapi* is actually our WILLPOWER.

Second we need to be mindful with full awareness of the object of mindfulness. We need to be fully aware of what is going on in the body and mind here and now. Instead of running on automatic pilot, we practice full awareness of what is happening in the present moment in a non-interfering manner. Compared to ordinary attention which is short and superficial, the attention in mindfulness is sustained, deep, full, and clear.

Third we need to comprehend and see things clearly and correctly. This third quality of clear comprehension is practically inseparable from mindfulness. When we are mindful, we will see things clearly. Seeing things clearly means seeing things as they are and not seeing things as what we believe they are, like seeing the body as the body and not seeing the body as the self, or seeing pain as pain and not seeing pain as suffering. Further elucidation of clear comprehension will be done in mindfulness of activities.

As we practice the first three components in sequence, the fourth which is removing greed and anger will occur as a result. First, we make effort to practice mindfulness. After a certain time when our mindfulness becomes firm and mature, we will be able to see things clearly. When we see things clearly, we are removing greed and anger from our mind or preventing them from arising. At every moment of practice of mindfulness, of practice of clear comprehension, we are removing greed and anger.

It is noteworthy to know that the order of the words in the teachings, i.e. ardent, clearly knowing, mindful, removing greed and anger, does not follow the sequence of the actual practice, the actual sequence is ardent, mindful, clearly knowing, removing greed and anger. In practice, we have to follow the order of the meaning, and not the order of the words. Effort comes first, followed by mindfulness, followed by clear comprehension, and then removing of greed and anger.

Definitions of mindfulness

Don't spend too much time in debating the various definitions of mindfulness. These definitions are merely modes of transport to the actual destination. If we want to go Kyoto, take a flight and go. Go and visit the magnificent Kiyomizu-dera wooden temple. Trek through the Arashiyama bamboo forest. Take a selfie at the Fushimi Inari Shrine in the evening light. And take a bite out of the gold-leaf Kinkaku ice-cream. If we spend a long time debating on the modes of transport, we may end up staying at home.

The four repeated instructions of *satipatthana*

Satipatthana Sutta: In regard to the body [feelings, mind and thoughts], one abides observing the body internally, externally and both. One abides observing the nature of arising in the body [feelings, mind and thoughts], the nature of passing away and both. Mindfulness that 'there is a body' [feelings, mind and thoughts] is established to the extent necessary for bare knowledge and continuous mindfulness. And one abides independently, not clinging to anything in the world.

These are the four instructions or refrains that are repeated thirteen different times in the teachings, following each of the specific mindfulness exercises. Refrain is a regularly recurring verse especially at the end of every stanza of a poem. I have counted these refrains a few times. There are thirteen refrains, one for each of the thirteen exercises in the teachings. In this book, we have more exercises than the actual thirteen exercises, but still in each exercise the instructions still apply. Through repetition of these instructions, we are reminded on the importance of these practices in establishing mindfulness.

First instruction, observing the body internally means paying attention to our own body [feelings, mind and thoughts]; and externally means the body [feelings, mind and thoughts] of others. Second, observing the nature of arising and passing away means paying attention to the changing nature of our experiences, the arising and passing away of our experiences. Third, bare knowledge means observing objectively without adding our own interpretations and stories, and continuous mindfulness means establishing mindfulness from moment-to-moment. Fourth, abiding independently without clinging to anything means paying attention without holding on tightly to any object. In the world means the respective field of practice – body, feelings etc.

The four mental qualities provide us four essential components in establishing mindfulness. The four refrains expand our scope of mindfulness practice spatially and temporally. We can say that the four refrains give us different levels of practice: from mindfulness of ourselves, to mindfulness of others, to both; from mindfulness of many moments of the arising 'now', to many moments of the falling 'now', to both. As for refining the quality of mindfulness, the practices of bare knowledge, continuous mindfulness, independent abiding and not clinging to anything prepare us to go deeper and deeper into our mind so we can one day see for ourselves the innermost essence of our mind – the unpolluted, pure, clear, radiant and brilliant awareness.

The four refrains of mindfulness

The four refrains are the PhD programme for mindfulness. It has a lot to do with research. We research our own mind and others'. We research the nature of arising and ceasing. We research with pure attention continuously, not clinging to anything.

A few final words before we go to the next chapter – mindfulness of the body. For the beginning, it is worthwhile to establish mindfulness with a technique called mental noting, which means the silent repeating of words or phrases such as "in", "out", "long", "short", "pleasure", "pain", etc., to support the continuity of mindfulness. Once our attention is strong enough, we can drop this technique to allow bare knowing to occur.

Right and wrong mindfulness

Mindfulness is an inborn quality of our mind. We all know what paying attention means. When I was a child I used to play in the field behind my house. During the rainy season, my brothers and I enjoyed watching the little tadpoles swimming around in the rain puddles. It was such a great fun just to see them wiggling. Sometimes we scooped them out and put them on the ground to watch them. But they died under the sun after a while. Watching the tadpoles dying on the ground is wrong mindfulness. Right mindfulness should at least do no harm to ourselves and others. At best, it should do good with a pure intention.

Mindfulness of the Body

Mindfulness of the breath (*Anapana*)

Mindful breathing is a beautiful spiritual practice. It is beautiful because it can bring a lot of joy to our life when we practice it. It is a spiritual practice because it can nourish the deepest core of our self. Mindful breathing involves paying continuous attention to breathing. If we think about a lot of things while we breathe, we are not really practicing mindful breathing. We are just breathing automatically, not mindfully. We are breathing absent-mindedly, not mindfully. We are absent-minded as far as breathing is concerned, but our mind may be full of everything else. For mindful breathing, we don't do that. We deliberately rest our attention on our breathing, not thinking about the past, present or future; but just breathe.

Mindful breathing means paying bare attention to breathing. When we breathe in, we know we are breathing in; when we breathe out, we know we are breathing out. We are aware of our breathing. We are aware of our breathing just as it is. We are not creating any stories for our breathing. We are also not creating any other stories in our mind. If we create a lot of stories in our mind, we are mind[full], not mindful. It means our mind is full, full of stories created by ourselves. But for mindful breathing, we are just interested in our breathing, nothing else. We just breathe.

To make it short, mindful breathing is breathing awareness. Continuous awareness describes the duration of mindfulness. We wish to stay mindful as long as we can, throughout the day, throughout our life. We may be interrupted by periods of mind[full]ness, but we do not blame ourselves. This is life. The modern society is like that. Everyone has a lot of things in their mind. Everyone is mind[full]. But that is ok. We just bring our attention back again and again to our breathing. It is a continuous practice, a lifetime practice. If we want to be mindful, we have to practice.

Bare awareness describes the quality of our mindfulness. Bare means we are only aware of breathing, nothing else. We are paying 100% attention to our breathing. Again, 90% of our attention may be occupied by something else. 30% may be our work. 30% may be our family. 30% may be entertainment. The modern society is a society of distractions. The more developed a country, the more distractions we have. But that is also ok. We just increase our attention again and again from 10% to 20%, 30%, 50%, 70%, 90% and finally 100%. When we lose our attention again, we do not have to blame ourselves. We just increase our attention to breathing back to 100%. We breathe, breathe, breathe, breathe, and breathe until our quality of mindfulness is 100%. This is mindful breathing.

Mindfulness itself is a kind of awareness. It is a kind of continuous awareness and bare awareness. Breathing is chosen to be the object of awareness because we breathe all the time. If we are alive, we will be breathing. We seldom stop breathing when we are alive. I can only think of a few exceptions. When we are very frightened by something, like if we see something climbing out from the television, we may stop breathing for a while. If we see someone very attractive, like when we meet Batman (Ben Affleck) or Wonder Woman (Gal Gadot) on the street, we may stop breathing for a bit longer. If we use the public toilet, we may stop breathing for as long as we are in the toilet. Other than that, we breathe all the time. Everyone breathes all the time. That is why breathing is chosen.

Breathing can act as a bridge that connects our body to our mind. Every time we remember we are breathing, our mind and our body will be one, working together, rather than working automatically and independently. When our mind and body are one, we can be grounded in the present moment. We can feel very at home, very comfortable. It is like after a long day work and we are finally back to home, sitting on the sofa, doing nothing. Can we imagine the feeling? It is very relaxing. When our mind comes home to our body, we can feel very calm and peaceful. It is like feeling home sweet home.

Mindful breathing acts as an anchor that keeps our attention at home. Without an anchor, our attention flies everywhere, all over the places. One moment we can be at the coffee shop. The next moment, our mind can fly to Venice riding the gondola. The next moment, we fly to Niagara Falls in Canada. Our mind has the tendency to fly everywhere, from one place to another, from one subject to another subject. That is why we need an anchor to keep our attention at home. Without this anchor, we will follow our imaginations, daydreaming and worries everywhere. We become servants of our imaginations, daydreaming and worries. We cannot become a master of our own mind. Our happiness and sorrow will be determined by others, by external circumstances. We lose control over our own happiness and sorrow. So, if we want to reclaim our control over our life, we have to reclaim our attention first. Not only we need to reclaim our attention, we need to keep it safely at home; so that we can use it whatever way we want, whenever we want, no longer being determined by circumstances. Then we can choose to move our attention from sorrow and stress to happiness and peace. And to reclaim our attention, the practice of mindfulness can be very helpful; to keep our attention at home, mindful breathing can be an excellent anchor.

We can practice mindful breathing according to our own schedule. In the beginning, we may start with 5 minutes every day. Then, we can increase the duration of the practice more and more. At the end, if we are ambitious, we may bring mindful breathing into our whole life throughout the day. Then, when we are ready, we can begin to share the practice with others who want to learn about it. I hope you can find a lot of joy in practicing mindful breathing. I hope you can develop lots and lots of happiness and peace from the practice of mindful breathing. So, happy breathing when you are reading this book!

Floaters and mindfulness

During those carefree childhood days I liked to lie on the long bench at the side of the football field and gazed at the clear blue sky. And I liked to play with the floaters. They looked like worms drifting in the air. Every time these worms fell slowly from the sky, I would bring them up again and again. Similarly, in mindful breathing, we bring our attention back to breathing again and again every time our attention drifts away.

It is important for us to develop a strong intention to practice mindful breathing before we start practicing. This intention is something like a wedding vow, like below:

I take my breath to be my husband/wife, my partner, my friend and my true love in life. I will cherish our companionship and love you more each day than the day before. I will walk with you, eat with you, laugh with you and cry with you, loving you faithfully through good times and bad, regardless of the obstacles we may face together. I give you my full attention, my heart and my love, from today forward for as long as we both shall live.

In order to sustain the practice of mindful breathing, we have to befriend our breath; we have to fall in love with our breath; and we have to marry our breath. We have to find joy while we are with our breath, during good times and bad times. Our breath has followed us from the first day of our life to now. It will continue to follow us until we take our last breath. We cannot find another friend who is that loyal. Our breath has given us life. And it is not expecting anything in return. Therefore, we have to start to treat our breath as our best friend. All we need to do is to give our breath a little bit more of our attention. Since to love is to be there, we have to be there for our breath.

Hawker stalls and mindfulness

I grew up in the small town of Gopeng where people knew each other in the neighbourhood. Every morning, we saw many hawker stalls lining up in front of the old shophouses at the High Street, selling a variety of goods and foods. I loved to frequent those stalls for traditional peanut pancake, sticky rice, Nyonya Kuih and so on. I could eat those foods again and again without getting bored not just because they were nice but also because the people there were friendly and they made me feel like we were one big family. What I ate was not mere food but also the human touch in the chunk of pancake, the lump of sticky rice and the small bite out of the Nyonya Kuih. In order for us to bring our attention back to our breath again and again like how I frequented those hawker stalls, we need to appreciate this human touch feeling in our breath so that we can stick to the practice no matter how short, long, peaceful or painful our breath is. Without this feeling, many people will stop practicing after a while when they get bored or distracted.

Back to intention, after developing a strong intention to practice mindful breathing, we still need to develop intention again and again every time we are practicing mindful breathing. It is often useful to divide the practice into a duration component and a quality component. For duration, it is about how much time we spend one day in the practice. For quality, it is about the depth of mindfulness that we are practicing.

Let us talk about duration first. Let us do some planning. Write down what we do in an ordinary day. We can get a diary, or a planner. Write down the daily events. Write down the sequence of events in one day – waking up, brushing teeth, washing hands, taking breakfast, driving to work, stopping at the traffic light, looking at the sky, walking to the office, talking to colleagues, having lunch, listening to patients, driving home, smelling flowers, going for exercise, having dinner, watching television, surfing internet, Facebooking, talking to family and sleeping. The list can be longer but I have cut it short. Break down our day into events. If we do not have time to write down the events, or we do not have enough money to buy a diary, we can just remember them in our mind.

As a start, we can develop the intention to practice mindful breathing just after waking up and just before going to sleep. These are two crucial moments that mark the beginning and the end of the day. A mindful beginning prepares us for mindful practices throughout the day. A mindful ending prepares us for the next beginning. After that, we can develop the intention to practice mindful breathing whenever we are free. It can be 1 minute, 3 minutes, 5 minutes or more. It can even be just one breath or two breaths if we are too busy. As time goes by, we can develop intention to practice mindful breathing with every daily event, one by one. Next, we can break down every event into a series of task. Then, we can develop the intention to begin and sustain the practice of mindful breathing during each task.

Take walking as an example; we can divide the event of walking into three tasks – lifting the foot, shifting the foot, stepping on the ground. As we progress, we may even break down each task into a stream of moments. These moments are small units of psychological time. Then, we can develop the intention to begin and sustain the practice from moment to moment. Forgive me if I sound a bit like a perfectionist. I am a perfectionist, minus the obsessive-compulsive part.

Developing the intention to practice mindful breathing is important because we tend to forget to practice. Sometimes we want to practice mindful breathing for a whole day but the moment we remember to practice, the whole day has gone. This is forgetfulness. Forgetfulness is a friend that gives us opportunity to practice. Every time we remember we have forgotten to practice, that is the beginning of a new practice. To add further, it is easier to focus on our breathing when we are alone. When we are with others, we may forget easily, especially so when we are talking to others or doing something with others. Therefore, we have to develop the intention to practice again and again every time we remember we have forgotten to practice. And we have to develop the intention to practice even when we are with others.

For quality, we need to slow down. The society now is a rushing society. This is very true if we are living in the cities. We can see everybody is walking very fast, like having a walking competition. Everybody has very little time. We have so many things to do. We just cannot stop moving. But this is not helpful when it comes to mindful breathing. To practice mindful breathing, we need to slow down first. Everything we do we do with a slower pace, but not too slow until everyone is looking at us. We slow down just enough for us to feel that we are not rushing. We slow down just enough for us to enjoy what we are doing. We walk slowly. We eat slowly. We drink slowly. We speak slowly. We drive slowly. We bathe slowly. But of course we do not slow down to the extent that we are causing problem to others, like my wife saying, "Hey! Have you finished bathing?" If someone is waiting for us, we need to speed up a bit without feeling rushed. If we cannot, then we rush mindfully. But at the beginning, rushing is not advisable. Once we are good in mindfulness, then rushing is not a problem.

Again it is about intention. We need to cultivate the intention to slow down again and again. We slow down to notice things that we may have missed so far in our day-to-day life – the fresh morning air, the fragrance of flowers, the smile of people that we meet, the swaying of trees, the falling leaves and so on. We slow down to appreciate our being more, and the beings of others. When we slow down we become more present for ourselves and others. We are like more alive. Then, we develop the intention to deepen our mindfulness practice again and again. From being mind[full], having a mind full of thoughts and feelings, we progress gradually to mindfulness, having one thing in mind at one time. From an expert of multi-tasking, doing many things all at once, we progress gradually to become an expert in uni-tasking, doing one thing at a time or even zero-tasking, doing nothing, simply be. Caution: Do not zero-task in front of your boss! I repeat. Do not zero-task in front of your boss! You may get fired.

To sum up, intentions are so important. Intentions to pay attention need to be repetitively cultivated. We need some effort in the beginning. With time, spontaneous intentions will arise. It is like eating ice-cream in a hot sunny day. We need some effort to make sure the ice-cream is not dripping. The pressure from our tongue needs to be just enough. Lick. Lick. Lick. And the ice-cream needs to be rotated from time to time. Once we become good in licking ice-cream, all of it will be caught by our tongue before it drips, effortlessly.

Mindful breathing and a little bit of neuroscience

As we breathe in and out, the sensation of airflow through the inside of our nose is detected by the nasociliary nerve and the nasopalatine nerve. These two nerves are branches of a larger nerve called trigeminal nerve. The trigeminal nerve carries the information of this nasal airflow sensation to a relay station called thalamus, which then projects the information to the sensory area of the brain (the primary somatosensory cortex). In the beginning of mindful breathing, the attention area of the brain (the anterior cingulate cortex) becomes active. As we continue to pay attention to our breath, our external awareness reduces, as represented by reduced activities of our visual and auditory areas of the brain; our internal chatter lessens, as shown by reduced activities of our language centre of the brain (Broca's and Wernicke's areas); our sensory pleasure and happiness increase, as shown by increased activation of the brain reward circuits (nucleus accumbens and medial orbitofrontal cortex). When our mindfulness deepens, activation of the attention area fades, followed by dimming of the reward circuits, eventually left with one-pointed attention to the object of mindfulness, allowing the brain to be extraordinarily calm to examine the minute details of all mental processes.

The first step of mindful breathing is to be aware of our own breathing. The awareness is essential. We can be breathing without awareness. But if we want to practice mindful breathing, we have to breathe consciously. Breathing in, we know we are breathing in. Breathing out, we know we are breathing out. It is that simple. Every time we breathe in, we pay attention to our breathing in. Every time we breathe out, we pay attention to our breathing out. When we notice that we are distracted by any sights, sounds, feelings or thoughts, we do not blame ourselves. We just gently bring our attention back to our breathing.

Now, try and see. Breathing in, we know we are breathing in. Breathing out, we know we are breathing out. Again, breathing in, we know we are breathing in. Breathing out, we know we are breathing out. If you find that the sentence is too long, you can try – breathing in, breathing out. Again, breathing in, breathing out. Breathe a few times and see. Can you do it? Breathing in, breathing out. Breathing in, breathing out. It is very simple. And it can be very calming. If we want it to be even shorter, we can try – in, out; in, out. Again, in, out; in, out. Every time we breathe in, we repeat the word 'in' slowly and silently in our mind. Every time we breathe out, we repeat the word 'out' slowly and silently in our mind. It has to be very silent so that it is not disturbing our attention on our in and out-breath. These words, phrases or verses are 'good friends' of mindful breathing. Whenever we are having a lot of thoughts or distractions, these friends will help us to focus more. Once we are not that distracted, we may continue with the practice without the help from these friends.

During the practice, we should allow the breath to happen naturally. We should not intentionally speed up or slow down our breath. We just follow our breath. We follow the breath entering our nose, passing through our windpipe, and reaching our lungs. Then, we follow it all the way out. We follow it in. we follow it out. We are like super fan of our breath. We may have a lot of followers in Facebook, Twitters, and Instagram etc. But for mindful breathing, we become the follower of our own breath. We try to follow our breath all the time. If we take 12 breaths a minute, we will breathe 720 times an hour and 17,280 a day. If we sleep 6 hours a day, then we will breathe 12,960 times during the day. Let us round it up to 13,000. Since every breath is a different breath, we aim to follow 13,000 breaths a day. We follow 13,000 in-breaths and 13,000 out-breaths. So, first of all, we aim to become a follower. Once we are good at following, we can call ourselves The Breath Follower. I am just kidding.

Following 13,000 breaths a day sounds impossible. But we do not need to worry. Among the 13,000 breaths, the most important one is this breath, not the last breath, or the next breath. It is this breath right now. Breathing in, we know we are breathing in. Breathing out, we know we are breathing out. Do you feel what I mean? Yes. This is great. The practice is to be aware of this breath right in the present moment. Breathing in. Breathing out. This breath. Not the last one. Not next one. Now, we are aware of our in and out-breath. Our attention has come back home thanks to the practice of mindful breathing. We can look around and see. Do you see things that you do not see before? Do you hear things that you do not hear before? Do you feel things that you do not feel before? No? It is ok. Continue you practice. Yes? Very good. Continue your practice.

Once our practice becomes more stable, we can choose a breathing reference point to narrow our focus of attention, such as the tip of our nose or mid-point between our tip of nose and upper lip. We establish mindfulness in front of us at that area. Then, we follow the entire length of the breath from the beginning, middle and end of the in-breath, to the beginning, middle and end of the out-breath. Breathing in a long breath, we know we are breathing in a long breath. Breathing out a long breath, we know we are breathing out a long breath. As our breath gets calmer, it will become shorter. Breathing in a short breath, we know we are breathing in a short breath. Breathing out a short breath, we know we are breathing out a short breath. With time, the breath will become smooth and harmonious. The flow of air will change from turbulent to laminar. Please take note that the long and short breath refer to the length of the breath, not the duration because for duration, it will change from short to long.

Then, we use our breathing to bring our mind back home to our body. And let the body and mind unite as one. Slowly, our body will calm down naturally. Breathing in, we feel our whole body when we are breathing in. Breathing out, we feel our whole body when we are breathing out. Breathing in, we feel the breath entering our body and calming all parts of our body. Breathing out, we let the breath takes away all our tension and tiredness.

So, let us start now with a few exercises on mindfulness of breathing. We can use these instructions of mindful breathing for ourselves, or use these instructions to guide others. There are four exercises of mindful breathing. We can start with one, then continue with the others when we have master one. Or we can practice all four in one go. It is up to you. Find one method that is most suitable for you. But here we will go through all four as an exposure for you.

Rainy days and mindfulness

My first home was a rented double-storey old shophouse at Kay Long Street, Gopeng. During rainy days, I liked to sit in front of the window upstairs and watched the rain fell down on the streets. There were so many things to watch, the rain, the puddles, the drain, the people, umbrellas, bicycles, motorbikes and cars. It was indeed a beautiful sight. I just need to be mindful of it.

Exercise 1: identifying the in and out-breath

- Go to a quiet place
- Sit down comfortably
- Fold or cross legs
- Or sit on a chair
- Sit upright
- Close our eyes gently
- Observe the breath at the nose area

- Breathing in, we know we are breathing in
- Breathing out, we know we are breathing out
- Do not control our breath in any way
- Just breathe naturally
- Do not be distracted by any thoughts
- Come back to our breath once we know we are distracted
- We can anchor our attention by silent mental noting like:
- In-out, in-out, or for Sanskrit's fans, "ana-pana", "ana-pana"
- Just be aware of the breath
- We are not interested in the last breath
- Not interested in the next breath
- But just this breath
- Breathe with full awareness of each in and out-breath

Exercise 2: following the entire length of the breath

- Make ourselves comfortable
- Close our eyes
- Follow the entire length of the breath: "the breath body"
- In-in-in-out-out-out, or "ana-ana-ana-pana-pana-pana"
- Do not allow any distracting thoughts to enter
- Breathing in a long breath, we know we are breathing in a long breath
- Breathing out a long breath, we know we are breathing out a long breath
- Breathing in a short breath, we know we are breathing in a short breath
- Breathing out a short breath, we know we are breathing out a short breath
- Do not force ourselves to take a long or short breath
- Just breathe naturally
- Just be aware of the entire length of the breath
- As we follow the breath, the breath will calm down naturally
- Breathe with full awareness of the entire length of the breath

Exercise 3: bringing our mind home to the body

- Use our breathing to bring our mind home to our body
- Stop ruminating about the past or worrying about the future
- Bring our mind back to the present moment
- Bring our mind and body together as one
- Breathing in, we are aware of our whole body
- Breathing out, we are aware of our whole body
- Mental noting: in-body-out-body, or "ana-kaya-pana-kaya"
- Feel the different parts of our body, from the top to the bottom
- Feel the body as a whole, fully united with the mind
- Feel the wholeness of ourselves with each breath

Exercise 4: calming the body

- Once our breath is harmonious, it will calm our body naturally
- Breathing in, we calm our body when we are breathing in
- Breathing out, we calm our body when we are breathing out
- Notice whether there is any tension in any part of our body
- Breathe and relax the tension one by one, from top to bottom
- Then relax the whole body all at once
- Feel the breath entering our body and calming all parts of body
- Feel the breath leaving our body and taking away our tiredness
- Mental noting: in-out-calm-smile-in-out-calm-smile

Satipatthana Sutta: Here, gone to the forest, or to the root of a tree, or to an empty hut, he sits down; having folded his legs, set his body erect, and establish mindfulness in front of him, mindful he breathes in, mindful he breathes out. Breathing in long, he knows he is breathing in long, breathing out long, he knows he is breathing out long. Breathing in short, he knows he is breathing in short, breathing out short, he knows he is breathing out short. He trains like this. He breathes in experiencing the whole body. He breathes out experiencing the whole body. He breathes in calming down his body. He breathes out calming down his body.

We can practice noticing our own breath, noticing the breath of others and noticing both. We can practice noticing the arising of the breath, the disappearing of the breath and both; noticing to the extent just enough to be simply aware of the breath from moment-to-moment; noticing to free ourselves from all the stories we create from time to time.

Mindfulness of postures (*Iriyapatha*)

The four main postures in our life are sitting, standing, walking and lying down. In mindfulness of postures, we pay attention to these four postures in a continuous manner. We pay attention when we change from one posture to another posture. The first posture of the day is usually lying down when we first wake up in the morning. This is our favorite posture. We usually want to remain lying down as long as possible in the morning, especially during rainy day. When we wake up, we can repeat the phrase "lying down", "lying down", silently in our mind. We can feel each contact points of our body with the softness of our bed. But don't practice this exercise too long or we will fall asleep again. Get up and sit at the edge of the bed and feel the contact of our soles on the floor. Then stand up slowly and walk.

Mindfulness of sitting is a useful practice we can do during our day. We can do it whenever we are sitting down. The first sit is usually at the breakfast table or the toilet bowl. Feel the contact between our body and the support. Feel the contact between our soles and the floor. We can also practice mindful sitting when we drive, when we sit at our office and when we come back home and sit at our sofa.

Toilet and mindfulness

Back in the 1970s, we used squat toilet in my grandparents' house. I had to be extraordinarily mindful while using it because there was a hole with a bucket below. First, I couldn't afford to slip and fall. Second, I had to keep my vision away from all the contents in the bucket. Third, someone might remove the bucket in the middle of my business time.

People always say don't just sit there, do something; but in mindful sitting, don't just do something, sit there! Sit like a mountain. Relax our body. Enjoy our sitting. If we can enjoy sitting in front of the television for hours, we should be able to enjoy mindful sitting too. The key is joy. Things that produce joy when we are doing it we can do it for a long time. So try and see whether we can bring an element of joy into our mindfulness practice.

Mindful sitting is best practiced during a traffic jam or a long-distance drive. We can pay attention to our breath, our body, our sitting and of course our surrounding too. Be aware of our body and contact points with the seat. Be aware of the beautiful sceneries all around us, if any. Be aware of other cars!

Mindfulness of standing can be practiced when we are brushing our teeth, washing our hands or talking to a friend while standing, but the best practice of mindful standing is when we are at a long queue. For example, when we are queueing up for Frozen Coca-Cola at Mc Donald, we can breathe in and out, and pay attention to our standing, the contact of our soles and the floor, the weight of our body and the movement when we shift forward little by little. We will have two rewards if we practice mindful queueing like this. Breathing. Breathing. Breathing. Standing. Standing. Standing. Queueing. Queueing. Queueing. We become more patient. And we get a cup of Frozen Coca-Cola.

Mindful walking can be practiced as we walk from one place to another. I love to practice mindful walking when I go to work. It is because there is a long corridor at the entrance of our faculty leading to the hospital, not because I want to be late to work. In mindful walking, we walk slowly. We walk and feel each step of our walking. We focus when we are lifting our foot, shifting it forward and placing it on the ground. We focus on the sensation when we move our body. We feel the clothes rubbing on our skin and the gentle wind caused by our movement. We walk in such a way as if we are calming down the earth. Walking. Walking.

Another place I love to practice mindful walking is at the night market. Taking a stroll at the night market can be very relaxing. We can walk slowly, paying attention to our walking and also the surrounding. We can feel the change of postures from standing to walking, or from walking to standing when we see something interesting or when we meet our friends there. Just walk slowly. Similarly, we can practice mindful walking during shopping but a word of caution, we may get enlightened if we practice mindful walking when we shop with our spouse. My wife can shop very long.

Exercise 5: awareness of postures

- Sit down comfortably
- Relax our body
- Pay attention to our sitting
- Notice the contact points of our body with the chair
- Bring our attention to our feet, our bottom and our back
- Notice the nature of our sitting posture
- Are we upright and relaxed? Are we tense? Are we slouching?
- Notice the different parts of our body
- Notice the intention to move our body
- Try to sit like a mountain
- Mental noting: sitting-sitting-sitting

- When we are ready, notice what we see in front and around us
- Notice what we hear right in the present moment
- At the same time, keep part of our attention on the sitting
- Then stand up slowly
- Pay attention to the change in postures from sitting to standing
- Pay attention to standing
- Feel our soles touching the ground
- Feel the minute vibrations and sways of our body
- Mental noting: standing-standing-standing
- Notice the different parts of our body while we are standing
- Again, notice the intention to move our body
- Be aware of what we see and hear around us while standing
- And when we are ready, we can go to a suitable place to walk
- When walking, we need to know we are walking
- We are not carried away by our thoughts and worries
- We are not rushing anywhere
- We just walk
- Pay attention to our feet as we step
- Stepping-stepping-stepping
- Feel the soles of our feet touching the ground
- Pay attention to our feet as we lift them up from the ground
- Lifting-stepping-lifting-stepping-lifting-stepping
- Feel the movement of lifting up and stepping down
- Pay attention to our feet as we shift them forward
- Lifting-shifting-stepping-lifting-shifting-stepping
- Enjoy the sensations of lifting, shifting forward and stepping
- Then drop the mental noting when we are ready
- And just pay attention to the whole process of walking
- Pay attention to the different parts of our body during walking
- Then, synchronize our breathing with our walking
- Breathing in, we lift our leg and move it forward
- Breathing out, we step on the ground
- Again, breathing in, we lift our leg and move it forward

- Breathing out, we step on the ground
- Again, breathing in, we lift our leg and move it forward
- Breathing out, we step on the ground
- Walk in a way to calm down our body and our mind
- Walking-walking-walking
- Calming-calming-calming
- Don't forget to smile while we are walking
- Smiling-smiling-smiling
- Now it is time to do our favourite practice – mindful lying down
- Lie down slowly on our yoga mat
- When lying down, we know we are lying down
- When lying down, we just lie down
- Feel the contact of our body touching the ground
- Feel the weight of our whole body
- Relax our whole body
- Let go of all tension in our muscles
- Lying down-lying down-lying down
- It is ok if we fall asleep, nobody is taking any picture
- It is safe to sleep here

Satipatthana Sutta: Again, when walking, he knows he is walking; when standing, he knows he is standing; when sitting, he knows he is sitting; when lying down, he knows he is lying down; or he knows accordingly whatever positions his body is located.

Again, we are encouraged to practice mindfulness of our own postures and the postures of others. We can sit at a crowded place like the food court and notice the different postures of others and the changes in postures. We can notice the arising of a new posture and the fading away of the old posture during changes in postures. Noticing these postures to the extent just enough to be simply aware of them from time to time; noticing how we are freed from all our mental fabrication when we pay complete attention to the bare experiences of these postures.

Mindfulness of activities (*Sampajanna*)

Of the four essential components of *satipatthana*, *sampajanna* is emphasized in mindfulness of activities. *Sampajanna* is translated as clear comprehension. It is related to four things: (1) Clear comprehension of the purpose of an activity. We have to ask ourselves. Is the purpose of the activity we are doing wholesome or unwholesome? Is the activity beneficial to us and others? Or is it harmful? Notice the possibility to choose a wholesome activity and abandon an unwholesome activity. (2) Clear comprehension of the appropriateness of an activity. Notice the appropriateness of an activity. Is it the right time and place to perform the activity? Are we with the right person to perform an activity together? (3) Clear comprehension of the fields of practice. We can ask ourselves. Which foundations of mindfulness are we practicing? Are we establishing mindfulness of the body, feelings, mind or thoughts? (4) Clear comprehension of the reality.

For clear comprehension of the reality, it is to be clearly aware of the three universal characteristics of reality. First is about the temporal reality that things change. Notice the big and small changes of every activity. Second is about the spatial reality that things are conditioned and impersonal. Notice the conditioning of an activity by the body, the sensations, the thoughts, the emotions and the consciousness. Don't take things personally. They are all conditioned by multiple factors. Third is about the psychological reality that things are unsatisfactory in nature. Notice the unhappiness when we cannot do things that we like and when we do things that we don't like.

The main message of clear comprehension is whether we are aware of the presence of stress or happiness when we are doing an activity. If we are doing an activity stressfully, then we are not doing it mindfully. In mindfulness of activity, we learn to enjoy everything that we do; we learn to do the right thing at the right time, right place and with the right person; we learn not to do wrong things that can harm us or others; and we learn to do things happily, with love, even for things as simple as opening and closing a door.

Opening door mindfully

Although we walk through many doors every day, not many of us make use of doors for the practice of mindfulness. The next time before we open a door, make full use of it to come back to the present moment. Breathe in and out. Stand straight. Feel our feet on the ground. Then lift our hand to hold the door knob. Turn it slowly. Breathe. Open the door. Breathe. Close the door. Listen to the sound of the door knob, and the door opening and closing. Look at the other side of the door. Take in the new scene, sound and smell. Be fully present when we open a door.

When we first wake up in the morning, we can remind ourselves how blessed we are because we are still alive! We can start our day with a kind wish such as wishing everyone to be happy. When we brush our teeth and change our clothes, we can pay full attention on brushing our teeth and changing our clothes. We can smile to ourselves when we look into the mirror. We need to take good care of our own body so that we can take good care of others later.

When we eat and drink, we can enjoy our breathing while waiting for the food. And feel grateful when the food arrives and say thank you to the person who serves us. And then we have to be there fully for the food. We can look at the food and smell our food for a while if nobody is watching. And put our food gently into our mouth when we are ready. Chew slowly. Feel the taste, texture and temperature of the food. Feel every nook and corner of the food. Feel the movement of the food as we chew and swallow. Follow the food down the foodpipe as we swallow and follow all the way down to the stomach. Feel the stomach for a while. And when we are ready, take the next portion of our food or take a sip of our drink. If we find ourselves thinking about our work or worries, gently come back to our meal. Do not eat our work and worries. Eat our food. Stop once we are full.

Exercise 6: mindful milo drinking

- Sit comfortably
- Relax our body
- Don't close our eyes for this practice
- Breathe in and out naturally if we haven't got our milo yet
- Spend a few moments feeling grateful
- Be grateful to Thomas Mayne from Australia who invented milo
- Be grateful to the person who serves us the milo
- Now look at the milo can
- Put it in our hand and feel it
- Shake it a little
- Then open it
- Smell it
- When we are ready, take the first sip, just a little
- Let the drink linger in our mouth for a while
- Taste it when it moves through the different parts of our mouth
- Taste it as if this is the last can of milo on earth
- Then swallow it and feel it flowing down your throat
- Feel it when it touches your stomach
- Optional: breathe out our milo breath through pursed lips
- And rest in the aftertaste in our mouth
- Repeat the steps for the next few sips
- And drink with full awareness of our drinking
- Be grateful for having milo to drink

For mindful bathing, before we bathe, make sure the door is locked. Then we can breathe in and out to center ourselves. Again look at the mirror and smile to ourselves. Take off our clothes slowly. For those of you with a great body, you can look into the mirror again but I normally just turn on the shower and bathe. Bathe slowly. Feel the contact and flow of the running water. Feel the temperature of the water. Wipe our body with soap. Feel the soap and the foam. We can play with the foam for a while like a child since nobody is watching us. Focus on the skin sensation when we put on the soap and wash it. If we find our mind wanders, come back to our sensation of bathing. Wash away all our worries, stress, and dirt. Rest our attention on the water showering all over our body. Turn off the shower. Wipe ourselves with a towel. Dress up nicely before we go out from the bathroom. This is mindful bathing. But please cut it short if someone is waiting outside to use the bathroom.

Same thing for any other daily activities in our life, we can always slow down and practice mindfulness of activities. Bring joy to every activity of our life, including our house chores. Some of us may not like the idea of housekeeping but in mindfulness of activities we practice joy even during housekeeping, such as sweeping, vacuuming or mopping the floor; preparing a meal, doing laundry or cleaning the toilet. We can smile a little when we are doing the housekeeping. We can practice mindful smiling when we are sweeping the floor. We just breathe in and out. Breathe in and out. And see our face as a flower bud. See. Not imagine. Choose any flower that we like. See the flower blooming slowly as we start to smile. Then smile very slowly until our smile is blooming fully. Rest our mind in the feeling of happiness. And let the feeling spread to our whole body as we breathe. Then start sweeping the floor!

Satipatthana Sutta: When going forward and returning he acts clearly knowing; when looking ahead and looking away he acts clearly knowing; when bending and straightening his limbs he acts clearly knowing; when wearing his clothes and carrying his bag he acts clearly knowing; when eating, drinking, consuming food and tasting he acts clearly knowing; when defecating and urinating he acts clearly knowing; when walking, standing, sitting, falling asleep, waking up, talking, and keeping silent he acts clearly knowing.

In this way, when we perform any activity we perform with clear comprehension. When we observe the activities of others we observe with clear comprehension. We recognize the arising and passing away of our experiences. Recognizing to the extent just enough to be clearly aware of the activity from time to time; abiding independently not clinging to anything in the world.

Mindfulness of the physical body

There is nothing wrong to take good care of our body. But we must understand that our body is subjected to disease, aging and death. No one can escape disease and death. Furthermore, our body is not as pure as it appears. It is full of impurities inside. The following exercise on mindfulness of the physical body helps us to become more aware of the impurities of our body and to become less attached to our body so we can let it go when it is time to let go. This practice deconditions our strong identification with our body that are, liking the superficial parts and disliking the deeper parts. We practice to lessen suffering that arises from this identification; and to reduce lust of all kinds, but not to produce disgust or hatred to our body. But if we find this section too challenging to practice, we may skip it. As for now, please continue to take good care of our body for ourselves and others.

Exercise 7: mindfulness of impurities (*patikulamanasikara*)

- Breathe in and breathe out
- Relax our body
- Review our body from the top of hair to the soles of feet
- Enclosed by skin
- Review our body as full of many kind of impurities
- In this body there are:
- Superficial parts: head hair, body hair, nails, teeth, skin
- Deep parts: fat, muscles, tendons, bones, marrow, diaphragm
- Solid organs: heart, lungs, liver, kidneys, spleen
- Hollow organs: stomach, bowels, mesentery
- Body fluid: bile, blood, lymph, pus, synovial fluid
- Excretion: tears, saliva, phlegm, mucus, sweat, urine, feces
- Notice the attractive and unattractive aspects of the body parts

The main purpose of this exercise is to help us to see our body parts as they actually are, without excessive attachment to the attractive parts and aversion to the unattractive parts. But if this is practiced repetitively with the wrong attitude, it can lead to disgust or hatred to our body. It may even lead one to commit suicide. The appropriate attitude is to see things just as they are without reacting to them. With the correct attitude, we can also practice this exercise to reduce our lust or hatred towards others. Just imagine looking inside the body of someone we love or hate. Review his or her thirty-one body parts one by one, secretly!

Satipatthana Sutta: Just as though there were a bag with an opening at both ends full of many sorts of grain, such as hill rice, red rice, beans, peas, millets, and white rice, and a man with good eyes were to open it and review it thus: 'this is hill rice, this is red rice, there are beans, these are peas, this is millet, this is white rice'; so too he reviews this same body.

*

Exercise 8: mindfulness of body composition (*dhatumanasikara*)

- Recognize the solid part of our body (the earth element)
- Feel the qualities of stiffness, hardness and softness
- Recognize the liquid part of our body(the water element)
- Feel the qualities of cohesiveness and fluidity
- Recognize the heat part of our body (the fire element)
- Feel the temperature of heat and cold
- Recognize the movement part of our body (the air element)
- Feel the qualities of extension, expansion and distension
- Notice the qualities of each element as we breathe
- Notice these qualities as we sit, stand, walk and lie down
- Notice these qualities as we perform our daily activities
- Notice similar elements that constitute the earth and universe
- Notice the interrelated nature of our body, earth and universe
- See our lives outside our bodies
- Transcend the boundary between self and nature
- Go beyond the limiting concepts of life and death

Working in the palliative care setting at some point we will be driven to reflect on our personal mortality. How ready are we to die? How do we want to die? What would be our reactions when someone we love faces death? What is our attitude towards death? How is our attitude towards death affecting our care of the dying patients? Nine points were suggested for the contemplation on death by the eleventh century scholar Atisha. Number one, death is inevitable. Two, our life span is decreasing continuously. Three, death will come, whether or not we are prepared for it. Four, human life expectancy is uncertain. Five, there are many causes of death. Six, the human body is fragile and vulnerable. Seven, at the time of death, our wealth is not useful to us. Eight, our loved ones cannot keep us from death. Nine, our own body cannot help us at the time of our death.

Death and my childhood

My earliest brush with death occurred when I was cycling down a slope in Gopeng Garden near my grandparents' new house. I was cycling so fast that I didn't notice a car coming from the left of a junction. I hit the car on its side. It screeched to a halt, dragging me along for a few meters. I was shocked but uninjured. If I cycled a little faster, I would have died. Death was so close to me. In fact, death has been following me all the time. So, it is better for me to make friend with him and learn from him as much as possible, especially about the preciousness of life. P.S. The driver followed me to my house and my grandmother paid him to repair his dented car.

Dying is almost always viewed as an unpleasant experience to everyone. We believe we will suffer when we die. We learn from our family and society how to respond to death and dying. It is something unpleasant and should be avoided and resisted, sometimes at all costs. We see dying as something that we do not like to go through or even think about. We deny that death and dying can happen to us. This is the main reason that when dying is actually happening, we grief, through many stages, as described by Elisabeth Kübler Ross in her book 'Death and Dying'.

Elisabeth Kübler-Ross described five stages of grief when one is dying. These stages are denial, anger, bargaining, depression and acceptance. When we are facing death, the first response can be a shock, followed by disbelief. Then, when dying continues, we may feel angry with what is happening. After that, we may start to ask for more time. But when things are not good despite our bargain, we will then sink into depression. May be only after a period of struggle, we may then begin to accept dying as a natural process that is useless to deny or fight against.

If we do not underestimate our human potentials, dying can indeed be a joyful journey. This cannot be achieved without some radical changes in our traditional mindset which is based on majority beliefs. But if one spends time on reflection of death and dying and begins to work on the preparation of dying, one can choose to view dying as a happy experience as opposed to our traditional beliefs. And when dying approaches, we can then experience dying in a joyful manner. This is a possibility that requires us to re-wire our brain radically. The notion of dying joyfully may sound radical but it is possible. Believe me.

First, dying joyfully begins with the acceptance of death and dying. On contrary of denying death and dying, this is represented by the full acceptance of dying with a curious mind. It includes the joyful acceptance of both pleasant and unpleasant experiences in dying, like acceptance of pain, loss of function, loss of body image, loss of dignity, loss of job, loss of roles, loss of friends, burdening family members, encountering uncaring healthcare staff and difficult moments in the hospital. This acceptance is marked by a curious and non-judgmental attitude. It is difficult to achieve this if we have not prepared our mind enough in letting go. But if we can achieve this, we will have bypassed all the initial four stages of grief – denial, anger, bargaining and depression.

After we have accepted death and dying, we can have a little planning now on how we want to die. What should we do for the rest of our life? What are our priorities in life? In what way should we live in order not to feel regret when we die? How can we live our life fully? How can we make our life more meaningful? We can work a little less and spend a little more time with our family and friends. We can go travelling every year. We can spend a longer time drinking our favourite drink or savouring our favourite food. We can lie down and rest without doing anything for an hour once a day. We can read more or pray more. Or we can explore what death actually is, mindfully.

If we prepare so, when dying arrives, we may feel excited or thrilled. Yes! Finally! It is our turn. We have prepared for our dying for such a long time and now it has arrived. It is time to have a first-hand experience now! I am not suggesting that we can savour pain and suffering but it is a common misunderstanding for one to think that the whole process of dying is ONLY pain and suffering. There are many moments of happiness and peace that many of us would have overlooked due to the lack of attention and the excessive focus on the negative aspects of dying. With complete acceptance of dying, we can start to savour our pain-free moments and do things that we enjoy. It can be simple things such as being with family, smelling a flower, reading books, looking out of the window or eating a piece of chocolate.

It is hard to believe that people can actually die happily. I have seen many happy deaths. People who are kind and contented tend to die happily. Some still can joke with us even though they are in pain. We can enjoy every precious moment that remains. We can do things that we still can do. And spend time with our loved ones. We can fill ourselves with a sense of delight no matter what is happening.

When all the excitement, happiness and delight are over, we may even feel a sense of inner peace. How should I describe this? It is like a great sense of relief after a celebration is over or after completing a great task. We can feel very carefree, peaceful and calm, unaffected by any intense emotions or negative thoughts. We may have some pain but we are no longer bothered by it so much. Happiness may arise but we feel like a peaceful observer, not greatly affected by it too. This state of calmness and equanimity prepares us for the final moments in life.

To achieve a joyful death, training in mindfulness can be helpful. We can prepare ourselves by practicing mindfulness of death. First, close our eyes. Relax our body. Breathe naturally. Be aware that death is a natural process in life. It can happen to us anytime, anywhere. Openly acknowledge that death can happen to us anytime, anywhere. Imagine we are dying and lying on a bed surrounded by our family. Feel the pain caused by organ failure. Experience the thoughts and emotions that arise. Watch them and let them be as they are without rejecting them. If fear arises, just breathe. If anger arises, breathe. If worry arises, breathe. If sadness arises, breathe and let go. Breathing in and out mindfully, we are at peace with death. Notice our breathing getting weaker and weaker. Smile a little. Then take our last breath.

Remember to breathe again after taking our last breath. It is just a practice. The practice of remembering death can be transformative. If we remember death, we will remember to live. We will see the preciousness of life. We will see the preciousness of time. We will see the preciousness of family and friends. And we will attach less to our wealth. To add, if we remember death in every breath, then we will remember to live, see the preciousness of life, of time, of family and friends, in EVERY breath.

Going one step further, we can practice mindfulness of the nine stages of the decomposition of a corpse. It is not a very pleasant exercise and is meant for those of us with good physical and mental health. But the result of this exercise can be liberating. It can liberate us from the excessive attachment to our body, knowing that it is just a corpse when we finally die.

Exercise 9: mindfulness of the corpse in decay (*navasivathika*)

- Lie down on our yoga mat again
- Close our eyes, breathe in and out, and relax our body

- Visualize a corpse in various stages of decay
- *Satipatthana Sutta*: As though we were to see a corpse thrown aside in a charnel ground – one, two, or three days dead, bloated, livid, and oozing matter... being devoured by crows, hawks, vultures, dogs, jackals, or various kinds of worms... a skeleton with flesh and blood, held together with sinews... skeleton without flesh but with blood ... skeleton without flesh and blood... disconnected bones scattered in all directions... bones bleached white, the color of shells... bones heaped up, more than a year old... bones rotten and crumbling to dust – we compare our same body with the corpse: 'our body too is of the same nature, it will be like that, we cannot escape it'

We can practice contemplating on our own impurities, body compositions, death and decomposition, contemplating on the impurities, body compositions, death and decomposition of others and contemplating on both; we can practice contemplating the phenomenon of arising in the body, the phenomenon of disappearing in the body, and both arising and disappearing; cultivating awareness to the extent just enough to be simply aware of the body in regard to impurities, body compositions, death and decomposition from moment-to-moment; abiding independently not clinging to anything in the world.

For some people, the most difficult practice is not to contemplate death and decomposition of their own body, but the death and decomposition of the body of their loved ones. It often evokes painful feelings that sometimes can be overwhelming. However, just like everyone else, our loved ones go through the same process of birth, aging, sickness and death too. Our loved ones will die too one day. This is a painful truth. The next section, mindfulness of feelings (*vedananupassana*) teaches us how to make use of feelings as an object of mindfulness.

Mindfulness of death

The moment we took our first breath, death was already there. If we don't die now, we will die later on. If we are not killed by an accident, we may die of a heart attack. If we don't die of a heart attack, we may die of cancer. If we don't die of cancer, we may still die of choking when we get old. Death is already there. When the time is up, we will die. If we see this, we will not suffer so much when we die. We must see this in order to truly live.

Mindfulness of Feelings

Introduction

Feeling in English can be a sensation, an emotion or an opinion. But the feeling in mindfulness of feelings is the translation of the Pali word *vedana*. It carries a more specific meaning. It refers to the feeling tone – the quality of pleasantness, unpleasantness and neutrality, which corresponds to *sukha*, *dukkha* and *upekkha* in Pali. These three feeling tones can be referred to as pleasure, pain and neutrality. They are the raw feelings underlying all sensations and emotions. These raw feelings deeply condition our habitual reactions and actions in our day-to-day life. To free ourselves from this deepest conditioning, *vedana* is a key factor.

To explain a little bit more about how *vedana* conditions our reactions and actions, we can first start with pleasure. When a pleasant feeling arises, we crave for the pleasant feeling (attachment reaction); and we try hard to seek the same pleasant feeling again and again (addictive behavior). As for pain, when an unpleasant feeling arises, we hate it (aversion reaction); and we try hard to resist it or avoid it (avoidance behavior). If the feeling is neutral, we are indifferent to it (ignorance reaction); and we don't care about it (couldn't-care-less behavior). This is how *vedana* conditions our reactions and actions.

All our live we have been chasing pleasure non-stop and also running away from pain. We have been running round and round in circle. This circle is called *samsara* in Pali. We are like an ox with its nose rings being pulled forward constantly by pleasure and whipped from the back by pain. So we cannot stop at all, going round and round, controlled by pleasure and pain.

Running away from pain

As far as running is concerned, I am exceptionally good. Everyone called my primary school tuition teacher Sister Twelve. I am not sure whether she is number twelve in her family or her name is literally Twelve. Her teaching strategy was to get us to memorize everything in our textbooks, including the instructions. I wasn't so sure how useful it was but never mind I just followed. We usually recited texts in small groups but I was late one day and she wanted me to do it alone. I wasn't very happy. So I sat on a chair for quite a while, keeping my eyes on my schoolbag, Then, in a flash I sprang to my feet, grabbed my schoolbag and sprinted through the door as fast as I could. Sister Twelve chase me from behind with her outstretched hand, shouting at me not to run away. It was a narrow escape, but as soon as my mother found out about the incidence I was brought back to the tuition center again. What a waste of my energy.

Practicing mindfulness of feelings helps us to recognize the transitory nature of feelings. It helps us to recognize our deeply ingrained habitual reactions to feelings, and not to objects. So we can have a choice to identify less with our feelings, to become less attached to pleasant feeling, less resistant to unpleasant feeling and less indifferent to neutral feeling. Mindfulness of feelings can make us less reactive and less judgmental. It helps us to foster a sense of calmness and equanimity.

But please don't get me wrong. I am not trying to say that we should avoid and resist pleasure and welcome pain and suffering. This is far from what I mean. There is nothing wrong to enjoy pleasure so long as we are not attached to it, so long we are not addicted to it, so long we can let go of it when we lose it or when we cannot get it. It is important to understand that happiness that comes from sensory pleasure is very unstable because of the transitory nature of feelings, and we need to repeat it again and again in an attempt to sustain it. In fact, it is not really sustainable because the greed for sensory pleasure can be insatiable.

So it is important to be aware of pleasure when it arises and disappears. The next time we eat ice-cream. Be aware of the pleasure when we are still holding it before we eat it. When we take the first bite, be aware of the pleasure from tasting it, the sweetness, the softness and the coldness. We can repeat the word 'pleasure', 'pleasure', 'pleasure' silently in our mind, or '*sukha*', '*sukha*', '*sukha*'. Witness the pleasure sensation migrates from the tongue to the mouth, the throat, the foodpipe and the stomach; and the pleasure from thinking about it. Notice the change in intensity of the pleasure from time to time. When we finish eating the whole thing, notice how pleasure disappears. And see what happens after that.

Kampung pleasures and mindfulness

Kampung is a local term for village. It is very easy to find simple pleasures from little things we do in Kampung. These little things are mostly free or you can say they are not really costly. In the morning, we have the nature alarm clock from different roosters. We have the smell of cool fresh air tinged with grassy scent. Neighbors greet us with smiling faces. And the list goes on – dry Wantan mee made according to a secret recipe, irresistible Ice Kacang and Rojak made by Auntie Japanese Doll, hugging huge water pipes on a hot day, wading across streams pretending to be a globe trekker, catching fighting spiders and so on. With a little mindfulness, it is not difficult to reclaim these Kampung pleasures in life, even while living in the city.

Similarly for pain I am not asking you to endure it or seek it deliberately. But the next time we experience pain, aside from taking the prescribed pain-killers, instead of trying to resist and fight against it, try to stay with it and see. Practice mindfulness of pain. Breathe in and out. Breathe until we feel calmer. Then bring our attention to the pain. We can say the word 'pain', 'pain', 'pain' slowly and silently in our mind, or '*dukkha*', '*dukkha*', '*dukkha*'. The focus should be on the unpleasant feeling but not the object that causes the feeling. Watch the pain arises when it arises. Watch it disappears when it disappears. Do not attempt to change it or reduce it. Just stay and observe the pain. If we notice the tendency to resist it, we try to relax this tendency. Smile to our pain and see what happens.

Although the teachings on mindfulness are separated into four foundations – the body, feelings, mind and thoughts, but the practices of mindfulness are all linked together. For example, when we practice mindfulness of the body, we need feelings to feel the body even though the focus is on the body. Focusing on the body in the beginning builds us a strong foundation for the second practice – mindfulness of feelings. Now, as we breathe, we can observe the feeling tone of our breathing. We observe how the feeling tone change when we breathe in an in-breath and when we breathe out an out-breath. Observe the degree or intensity of the feeling tone as we breathe in and out.

Then, observe the feeling tone of the entire length of the in and out-breath. Observe the feeling tone of our whole body. Observe the feeling tone of our whole body as it calms down. After that, we can practice mindfulness of feelings of our four postures and our daily activities. Observe our feelings as we sit, stand, walk and lie down. Observe our feelings as we carry out our daily activities.

Similarly, we can practice observing our feelings when we review our bodily impurities and body composition; and when we contemplate death and the decomposition of corpse. The reason why *vedana* is the key factor to liberate us from suffering is because it is a crucial step in the formation of suffering. When we see a person we hate, first an unpleasant feeling arises, the no good feeling, the *dukkha* feeling, but up to this point the experience is still pure, there is still no suffering. Suffering arises when we start to react to this feeling of unpleasantness, like 'I don't like you' or 'I don't want to see you'. Then a story will be created by ourselves about this person we hate, followed by actions and behaviors such as quarreling with the person or walking away from the person.

Up until the point of feelings the experience is still pure, but as soon as we react then suffering arises. The actual psychological processes of suffering formation comprise (1) contact (*phassa*) – the meeting of senses and sensory objects or the meeting of the mind and mental objects, (2) feelings (*vedana*) – the arising of feelings because of contact, (3) craving (*tanha*) – the reactions of attachment, aversion or ignorance towards the three feeling tones, (4) clinging (*upadana*) – the persistence of attention and reactions on the feelings, creating a story or multiple stories, sometimes we can write a book from these stories, and (5) birth (*jati*) – the birth of action, the running towards pleasure and running away from pain.

So, for mindfulness of feelings, when *sukha* arises, we note it, *sukha, sukha, sukha*. When *dukkha* arises, we note it too, *dukkha, dukkha, dukkha*. When *upekkha* arises, we say *upekkha, upekkha, upekkha*. If our mindfulness is strong, then there will be no room for reactions. If we practice for a whole day, our whole day will be *sukha, sukha, dukkha, upekkha, upekkha, sukha, sukha* and so on.

Gross psychological processes
(Without mindfulness)

Perception
(Becoming aware of a sensory object)

↓

Reactions
(Cognitive, emotional and behavioural reactions)

Microscopic psychological processes
(With mindfulness)

Contact
(The meeting of senses, sensory objects and consciousness)

↓

Feelings
(The arising of feeling tones)

↓

Craving
(The reactions towards the three feeling tones)

↓

Clinging
(The persistence of reactions)

↓

Birth
(The birth of actions and behaviour)

Quantum psychological processes
(With advanced mindfulness)

<u>Seventeen moments of psychological processes</u>

*Interruption of bhavanga**

Sensory object enters sense organ
↓
Vibration caused by signal transduction
↓
Flow of consciousness interrupted
↓
Perception

Consciousness turning towards senses
↓
Consciousness meeting the sensory object
↓
Consciousness receiving the sensory object
↓
Consciousness investigating the sensory object
↓
Consciousness determining the sensory object
↓
Reactions

Seven moments of *javanas***
↓
Storing of experiences in two moments

*bhavanga – the flow of consciousness when there is no thoughts
**javana – the reactions of the mind towards the sensory object

Exercise 10: identifying the feeling tone

- Make ourselves comfortable
- Relax our whole body
- Breathe naturally
- Observe the feeling tone of our in and out-breath
- Is it pleasant, unpleasant or neutral?
- Observe the feeling tone from moment-to-moment
- How does our feeling tone change as we breathe in and out?
- How does our feeling tone change from moment-to-moment?
- One moment is called *khana* in Pali
- 1 second ≈ 75 moments (*khana*)
- 1 breath ≈ 100-400 moments or more
- How many moments of feeling can we observe in one breath?
- It is ok if we can just observe 3 moments, or 5 moments, or 10
- Pay attention to the arising and disappearing of the feeling tone
- Do not attempt to control or change the feeling tone
- If we are distracted, return our attention to the feeling tone
- Feeling a pleasant feeling, we know we are feeling a pleasant feeling
- *Sukha, sukha, sukha* ...
- Feeling an unpleasant feeling, we know we are feeling an unpleasant feeling
- *Dukkha, dukkha, dukkha* ...
- Feeling a neutral feeling, we know we are feeling a neutral feeling
- *Upekkha, upekkha, upekkha* ...
- Observe the tendency to crave for a pleasant feeling
- *Vasana, vasana, vasana* (habitual tendency) ...
- Observe the tendency to hate an unpleasant feeling
- *Vasana, vasana, vasana* (habitual tendency) ...
- Observe the tendency to ignore a neutral feeling
- *Vasana, vasana, vasana* (habitual tendency) ...
- Notice the suffering that arises from resisting painful feeling
- Notice the suffering that arises from craving pleasant feeling

- Try not to react towards any feeling tone
- Give ourselves some space to see how best to respond
- Contemplate impermanence in those feelings
- Let the feelings come when they come
- Let the feelings stay when they stay
- Let the feelings fade away when they fade away
- Watch the feelings come, stay and fade away
- Do not cling to any feeling
- When we do not cling to any feeling, we are not agitated
- When we are not agitated, we are free from stress

Exercise 11: identifying the source of the feeling tone

- Sit comfortably
- Relax our whole body
- Look around us
- Look closely
- Take in everything we can see
- Observe the feeling tone of our seeing
- Notice the source of the feeling tone
- Is it from the body or from the mind?
- Now close our eyes
- Pay attention to our hearing
- Take in everything we can hear
- Observe the feeling tone of our hearing
- Notice the source of the feeling tone
- Is it from the body or from the mind?
- Sniff the air in front of us
- Observe the feeling tone of our smelling
- Notice the source of the feeling tone
- Is it from the body or from the mind?
- Wiggle our tongue a little
- Observe the feeling tone of our tasting
- Notice the source of our feeling tone
- Is it from the body or from the mind?

- Now pay attention to our sitting posture
- Observe the feeling tone of our sitting
- Notice the source of the feeling tone
- Is it from the body or from the mind?
- Now pay attention to our different body parts one by one
- Observe the feeling tone of different parts of our body
- Head, neck, chest, upper limbs, abdomens, lower limbs, soles
- Are the feeling tones of different parts all the same or different?
- Notice the source of the feeling tone
- Is it from the body or from the mind?
- Now think about something we like
- Then think about something we don't like
- Observe the feeling tone of our thoughts
- Notice the source of the feeling tone
- Is it from the body or from the mind?
- Now, breathe in and out slowly
- Bring our attention back to the present moment
- Come back to all our senses and mind as a whole
- Observe the overall feeling tone
- Notice the source of the feeling tone
- Is it from sight, hearing, smell, taste, touch or thoughts?
- We can label the feelings *sukha, dukkha, upekkha*
- We can also label the source, *kaya* (body), *citta* (mind)
- Example: pleasure-body → *sukha-kaya*
- Example: pain-mind → *dukkha-citta*
- Observe our feeling tone when we carry out our daily activities
- Notice the changes in feeling tone
- Notice the changes in the sources of the feeling tone

The best way to practice mindfulness of feelings in our contemporary society is to go and watch a movie. Observe the different feeling tones that arise and fade away while we are watching it. It can be a comedy, a love story, an action movie or a horror movie. Just pay attention to our changes in feeling tones in different types of movies. *Sukha, sukha, dukkha, dukkha, upekkha, upekkha.* When we watch a comedy, it is mostly *sukha, sukha, and sukha.* When we watch a horror movie, it is mostly *dukkha, dukkha and dukkha.* When we watch a love story, it will be *sukha, dukkha, sukha, dukkha.* When we watch a boring movie, it will be *dukkha, dukkha, upekkha, upekkha.* Observe our tendencies of craving a pleasant feeling, hating an unpleasant feeling or feeling 'meh' for a neutral feeling. Feeling 'meh' means indifferent. I learnt this word after watching the movie Emoji.

When we go a little further, we can divide feelings into worldly and unworldly feelings. Worldly is *samisa* in Pali. It means that which arises from the flesh. Worldly feelings refer to feelings that arise from our senses and our mind that are associated with the tendencies of craving, hating or ignoring. Examples are sensory pleasure (worldly pleasant feeling), physical pain (worldly unpleasant feeling) and indifference (worldly neutral feeling).

Unworldly is *niramisa* in Pali. Unworldly feelings refer to feelings that are not associated with the tendencies of craving, hating and ignoring. Examples are happy feeling that results from spiritual practices such as giving without expectation, loving without conditions; and happy and unhappy feelings that arise from practicing renunciation, mindfulness and meditation (unworldly pleasant and unpleasant feelings). The feeling of equanimity during the practice of mindfulness and meditation is an example of unworldly neutral feeling.

Exercise 12: identifying worldly and unworldly feelings

- Think of a time when we feel happy
- Is our happiness associated with any selfish desire?
- Is our happiness associated with any dissatisfaction?
- Is our happiness associated with any absentmindedness?
- If it is, it is a worldly pleasant feeling

- Think of a time when we feel happy after helping someone
- Is our happiness associated with any selfish desire?
- Is our happiness associated with any dissatisfaction?
- Is our happiness associated with any absentmindedness?
- If it is not, it is an unworldly pleasant feeling
- Think of a time when we feel happy after loving someone
- Is our happiness associated with any selfish desire?
- Is our happiness associated with any dissatisfaction?
- Is our happiness associated with any absentmindedness?
- If it is not, it is an unworldly pleasant feeling
- Observe every feeling when it arises
- Observe whether it is a worldly or unworldly feeling
- Observe whether any tendency is present
- Recognize the tendency to chase worldly pleasant feeling
- Recognize the tendency to resist worldly unpleasant feeling
- Recognize the tendency to ignore worldly neutral feeling
- Let these tendencies be as they are without increasing them
- Recognize the absence of tendency in the unworldly feelings
- Appreciate and cultivate the unworldly feelings
- We may use the following mental noting
- *Samisa sukha vedana* – worldly pleasant feeling
- *Samisa dukkha vedana* – worldly unpleasant feeling
- *Samisa upekkha vedana* – worldly neutral feeling
- *Niramisa sukha vedana* – unworldly pleasant feeling
- *Niramisa dukkha vedana* – unworldly unpleasant feeling
- *Niramisa upekkha vedana* – unworldly neutral feeling

To recapitulate, feeling tone experiences an object directly, like a king enjoying his meal as much as he likes; compared to other thoughts that experience the object indirectly, like the cook who prepares the dish for the king and he only gets the chance to sample the food while preparing it.

Because feeling tone experiences objects directly, it provides us with quick feedback that conditions our reaction and action. In dangerous situation like when we are being chased by a buffalo, this split-second reaction and action can be life-saving. But in the relatively safe situation right now, at least for most of us, since we hardly see any buffalo roaming the streets, this survival function of feeling tone can sometimes produce inappropriate reactions.

So, it can be useful to practice mindfulness of our feelings to be aware of how we are conditioned by our feeling tones, and how society and commercials make use of this understanding to condition our habits of spending and living, consciously or subconsciously. It is about time to make a list of our bad habits and be mindful of the conditioning of our reactions and actions by our feelings. Try to change our bad habits by looking deeply into the conditioning of them. And cultivate good habits such as practicing mindfulness!

Satipatthana Sutta: In this way, in regard to feelings he abides observing feelings internally... externally... internally and externally. He abides observing the nature of arising... of disappearing... of both arising and disappearing in feelings. Mindfulness that 'There is feeling" is established in him to the extent necessary for bare knowledge and continuous mindfulness. And he abides independent, not clinging to anything in the world.

Tsunami and unworldly feelings

When Tsunami hit Aceh in 26th December 2004, hundreds of thousands of people were injured and killed. 100 million became homeless. I cried silently *(unworldly painful feelings)* while I was watching a late night Hong Kong charity show doing fundraising for Aceh. It was so much pain to watch those people affected by the tragedy. So I sneaked into my room while my wife was still sleeping and took out all my coins from a jar. The next day, I went to the bank and took out all my savings. I gave them all to Tzu Chi Foundation for disaster relief. I gave away all my money that day for a good reason and I felt so happy about it. In fact, every time I think about the experience I feel very happy *(unworldly happy feelings)*.

Mindfulness of Mind

Introduction

The third foundation of mindfulness is mindfulness of mind. The Pali word for mind here is *citta*. *Citta* means a process of thinking or knowing an object. Unlike mindfulness that is fully aware of an object, *citta* is just a form of simple awareness of an object. This awareness of an object is always accompanied by thoughts (*cetasika*), like bad thoughts such as greed, anger and ignorance; or good thoughts such as generosity, kindness and mindfulness.

Citta can be considered as the leader of thoughts. It controls them and is always accompanied by them. When the mind is accompanied by good thoughts, we call it the wholesome mind (*kusala citta*); when it is accompanied by bad thoughts, we call it the unwholesome mind (*akusala citta*).

To start with, mindfulness of mind is practiced by observing whether our mind is wholesome or unwholesome. It means to observe all our positive and negative mental states. All negative mental states can be broadly classified into three – greedy mind (*raga*), angry mind (*dosa*) and ignorant mind (*moha*). Likewise, all positive mental states can be classified into three – non-greedy mind (*araga*), non-angry mind (*adosa*) and non-ignorant mind (*amoha*).

As we experience a pleasant feeling, as soon as we crave for the pleasant feeling, the greedy mind arises. As we experience an unpleasant feeling, as soon as we resist the unpleasant feeling, the angry mind arises. As we experience a neutral feeling, as soon as we ignore the feeling, the ignorant mind arises.

Up to the level of feelings, the mind is still pure, but as soon as we react to the feelings, it will be polluted by greedy, angry or ignorant thoughts. The pollution is there, but the nature of mind is always free and spacious. In mindfulness of mind, we observe the presence or absence of these pollutions; and more importantly, we observe the quality of our mind when it is polluted and when it is not. This is for us to recognize that the nature of our mind is intrinsically free from these three polluting thoughts, which means the three unwholesome thoughts are not inherent and they are not the nature of the mind itself. They are the byproducts of the mind!

On a subtler level, the greedy mind and the angry mind can be called the 'I want'-mind and the 'I don't want'-mind. Although not everything that we want or don't want is unwholesome, but it is worthwhile recognizing the driving forces of these two states of mind as far as freedom is concerned. When we lose something we want or we cannot get something we want, we suffer. When we gain something we don't want, we suffer too. Notice the freedom from suffering when we are free from 'I want' and 'I don't want'.

As for the ignorant mind, it is actually the root cause of both the greedy and the angry mind. It can be called the 'I'-mind. It is not the 'I' in I-pad and I-phone, but the 'I' in 'I want' and 'I don't want'. When the mind is ignorant, it is unaware. Number one, it is unaware that lasting happiness is not achieved through avoiding pain and pursuing sensory pleasure because pain is inevitable in life and pleasure is transient. That is why the 'I'-mind continues to chase pleasant feeling with the 'I want'-mind and chase away unpleasant feeling with the 'I don't want'-mind. It is unaware that lasting happiness is achieved through abandoning the greed for sensory pleasure and relaxing the resistance for pain, quite the opposite from what the 'I'-mind is doing all the time!

Number two, the 'I'-mind is unaware that nothing lasts; therefore it tries to hold on to things that it likes and avoid things that it doesn't like, but of course futilely. Number three, it is unaware that the 'I' that it cherishes so much is just a mental construction based on its body, feelings, thoughts, emotions and consciousness. Therefore, recognizing these three unwholesome mental states and the absence of them may be the answer that frees us from our cyclical movement (chasing pleasure, chasing away pain) of existence.

The practice of mindfulness of mind is not an easy job. When we practice mindfulness of the body we can feel our body, it feels real. When we practice mindfulness of feelings we pay attention to our feelings, they are there. But the mind can be everywhere, from here in the room to as far away as one of the distant corners of the universe or beyond, from now in the present moment to the history of our long gone past and our dream-like future that is not yet here.

So I suggest we keep our attention on our breath and watch our mind from a distance. The mind is like the little sparrows skittering in front of my house. I can watch them from a distance behind my glass door but as I approach them they will fly away. If I feed them and then hide myself, they will come again. This is similar to practicing mindfulness of mind, watch from a distance, and we will see all the different types of birds that come after we spread the seeds on the ground.

As we see greedy, angry or deluded birds, we stop feeding them. They will fly away by themselves. We don't have to chase them away. As we see good birds like kind, caring or happy birds, we feed them and let them stay longer. But we must understand they don't stay forever. That is why it is more important to be aware when there is no bird. The mind will be clear and free.

Exercise 13: identifying unwholesome/wholesome mental states

- Now we are going to do an interesting exercise
- It is called catching the mind
- Unlike the body which is tangible, that we can touch it
- And unlike the feelings which are so close to our body
- Mind is pretty hard to catch
- I can reassure you that it is harder than catching birds
- That is why we start with mindfulness of the breath
- When we are grounded, then we are ready to catch our mind
- Now let our mind wanders without trying to control it
- Let it wander wherever it wants to go
- It can wander to the past or future
- It can stay at the body or travel to the distance
- Just let it wanders
- Do not try to chase it
- We won't be able to chase it because our mind is very fast
- Do not try to chase it away either
- Our mind can run faster than us
- Just stay with our breathing
- And observe our mind running around
- Then, out of a sudden, take a snapshot of our mind
- See whether we can catch any unwholesome mind
- Is it a greedy mind, angry mind or ignorant mind?
- Is it an 'I want'-mind, 'I don't want'-mind or 'I'-mind?
- It is ok if we fail to catch one after some time
- Then just bring one into our mind
- Imagine when we open our fridge and see all our desserts there
- Then catch our greedy mind
- Notice the arising of the greedy mind
- How does a greedy mind feel like?
- Observe the greedy mind without reacting to it
- *Raga-raga-raga*
- Observe until the greedy mind fades away
- Recognize that the greedy mind has gone

- Reflect on the nature of a greed-free mind
- *Araga-araga-araga*
- Is it free, happy, generous, loving and compassionate?
- Now imagine when we are quarrelling with someone
- Then catch our angry mind
- How does an angry mind feel like?
- Notice the arising of the angry mind
- Observe the angry mind without reacting to it
- *Dosa-dosa-dosa*
- Observe until the angry mind fades away
- Recognize that the angry mind has gone
- Reflect on the nature of an anger-free mind
- *Adosa-adosa-adosa*
- Is it free, happy, relaxed, peaceful and friendly?
- Now about ignorance
- The mind is clear and aware before ignorance arises
- Now think about 'I', like 'I am the best'
- Notice the arising of the ignorant mind
- *Moha-moha-moha*
- Once we pay attention, the ignorant mind fades away
- Recognize the re-appearance of the clear and aware mind when our mindfulness if strong
- Recognize the nature of an ignorance-free mind
- *Amoha-amoha-amoha*
- Is it clear, aware, spacious and bright?

Satipatthana Sutta: Here one knows a greedy mind to be 'greedy', and a mind without greed to be 'without greed'. One knows an angry mind to be 'angry', and a mind without anger to be 'without anger'. One knows an ignorant mind to be 'ignorant', and a mind without ignorance to be a mind 'without ignorance'.

Passive wholesome mental states

In 1998, I did my elective posting in Hualien Tzu Chi Hospital in Taiwan. The experience was one of the happiest in my life. People there were so nice and friendly, treating me like their family. My batchmates and I went travelling every weekend. The sceneries were amazing. We went to places such as Taroko National Park, Mount Hehuan, Qingjing Farm, Wuling Farm, East Coast and Kenting National Park. We also stayed at the Abode of Still Thoughts to experience the peace of monastic life. After coming back from Taiwan I felt an undescribable sense of peace. I was free from all stress for many months. The peace was caused by external circumstances. But I can't reproduce that same sense of peace up until I started to practice mindfulness a decade later.

If we find that catching the three types of unwholesome mind and the three types of wholesome mind too tiring. Then, just catch the thinking mind first. Just note it silently in our mind, thinking, thinking, thinking, or *citta, citta, citta*. Does it sound easier? If yes, we can continue with this simple practice first. Thinking, thinking, thinking. If we are focusing on our breath, once our mind wanders, we just note it. Wandering, wandering, wandering. Then come back to our breath. This is the practice of mindfulness of mind.

Another way to practice mindfulness of mind is to scroll our Facebook or Instagram and observe our mind. Number one, are we craving for an attractive picture of food, person, scenery or post? Is our mind greedy? Are we feeling upset for a negative picture or post? Is our mind angry? Or are we scrolling down aimlessly? Is our mind ignorant? Number two, for our own photos and posts, are we craving for more likes and positive comments? Are we feeling upset with little likes and negative comments? Or are we uploading a picture or post without knowing its potential consequences on ourselves or others?

Since some of us spend so much time in social media it can be very useful to make full use of these social media apps for the practice of mindfulness. We can also be mindful the next time our hand is reaching for our phone. What triggers us to reach for our phone? What is in our mind when we reach for our phone? Any craving? Any dopamine release? Is it just another conditioning?

Once we are good in identifying the unwholesome and wholesome mind, we can then practice identifying the eight pairs of mind. Observe whether our mind is greedy or not greedy; angry or not angry; ignorant or not ignorant; drowsy or restless, narrow or wide; concentrated or not concentrated; deeply concentrated or not deeply concentrated; and free or not free.

A greedy mind feels like it is burning with the fire of craving; a not greedy mind is calm, cool, peaceful and relaxed. An angry mind is gripped by anger or hatred; a not angry mind is calm, cool, peaceful and relaxed. An ignorant mind is stubborn, inflexible and full of cognitive errors; a not ignorant mind is calm, cool, peaceful, alert, clear and free.

A drowsy mind is dull and heavy, collapsing inward; a restless mind is agitated and hyperactive, expanding outward. A narrow mind is limited and restricted; a wide mind is vast and spacious. A concentrated mind is focused; a not concentrated mind is unfocused. A deeply concentrated mind is deeply focused; a not deeply concentrated mind is not deeply focused. A free mind is free from all problems, not greedy, not angry and not ignorant, spacious and deeply focused; a not free mind is bound by problems, greedy, angry or ignorant, restricted and unfocused.

In this way, in regard to the mind we can observe our own mind, the mind of others and both. We observe the nature of arising, of fading away, and both in regard to the mind. Mindfulness that 'There is a mind' is established to the extent necessary for bare knowledge and continuous mindfulness. And we abide independently not clinging to anything in the world.

Instant mindfulness

In 2008, I read a book called The Joy of Living by Yongey Mingyur Rinpoche. From the writings, I was introduced to the secrets of finding joy and happiness in everyday life. After reading the book, I started to meditate 5 minutes every day. I started with mindful breathing. And as I began to taste the benefits of my practice, I increased the duration of my mindful breathing to 20min, 30min, 45min or even 1 hour. As time went on, I continued to explore the different types of mindfulness meditation from reading. Then, I extended my practice from mindful breathing to mindful walking, mindful eating, mindful driving, mindful bathing and so on. A few months later, I noticed my stress disappeared completely. I felt the same sense of undescribable peace that I experienced when I was in Taiwan but this time it was an internal thing, happened particularly after each mindfulness practice. Stress still occurs once in a while but as soon as I remember to be mindful, as soon as I come back to the present moment, it disappears very rapidly. Now, I realize that whenever we experience a stressful situation, if we can remain mindful, the stress will disappear instantly. It is like instant mindfulness. The feelings may linger for a while. But the stress disappears instantly. In the current fast-paced society, we need more instant mindfulness. With instant mindfulness, we can easily add other ingredients to our mind whenever we want, such as instant gratitude, instant contentment, instant happiness and instant love; even when we are eating instant noodles.

Mindfulness of Thoughts

Introduction

The fourth foundation of mindfulness is mindfulness of *dhamma*. The Pali word *dhamma* carries a wide range of meanings, such as law, reality, teachings, but here it is best referred to as thoughts. Five categories of thoughts are described in mindfulness of thoughts. They are the five hindrances, the five aggregates, the six sense-spheres, the seven awakening factors and the four noble truths. The first three categories involve observing thoughts that block psychological freedom, and the last two categories involve observing thoughts that lead to psychological freedom.

Mindfulness of the five hindrances (*nivarana*)

The five hindrances are the five types of thoughts that hinder the progress of mindfulness practices. They are the **distractions** of practices. These five hindrances are liking, disliking, drowsiness, restlessness and doubt. The nature of our mind is like clear water. But when hindrances are present, the water will be disturbed.

When liking, desire or greed (*kamacchanda*) is present, it is like water with all the colorful dyes in it. When disliking, anger or hatred (*byapada*) is present, it is like hot boiling water, bubbling constantly. When drowsiness, dullness or laziness is present (*thina-middha*), the water is stagnant and stale, with algae, moss and slime growing on the surface. When restlessness or worry (*uddhacca-kukkucca*) is present, the water is like being whipped up by the wind, with lots of ripples and waves. When doubt (*vicikiccha*) is present, the water is murky, like a cloudy suspension placed in a dark room. With the hindrances, we cannot see our mind clearly.

Let us look at a few examples to understand the hindrances better. Imagine we are sitting and practicing mindful breathing. Suddenly we think about eating ice-cream. That is a liking hindrance. We want to eat Haagen-Dazs ice-cream. When we practice mindfulness of thoughts, we repeat 'liking', 'liking', 'liking' silently in our mind. Just observe the thoughts of liking without reacting to them. If we think we cannot sit anymore, this practice is so boring. That is a disliking hindrance. We can repeat 'disliking', 'disliking, 'disliking' silently in our mind. Just observe the thoughts of disliking without reacting to them.

Even if we are drowsy, we can be mindful of our drowsiness and say 'drowsiness', 'drowsiness, 'drowsiness'. If we are tired, say 'tiredness', 'tiredness', 'tiredness'. If we are lazy, say 'laziness' only once since we are lazy. Just kidding. If we are restless, just say 'restlessness', 'restlessness'. If we are worried, say 'worry', 'worry'. If we are stressed, say 'stress', 'stress'. If we have doubt or confusion, say 'doubt', 'doubt', or 'confusion', 'confusion'.

We need to know that the real problems come when we are not aware of hindrances and we recycle these hindering thoughts. When we think about an ice-cream we start to think about it again and again. Instead of focusing on the hindrance of liking we focus on the ice-cream. And we create a whole story of ice-cream.

When we are angry about someone, the problem comes when we continuously think about the person who makes us angry. Instead of being mindful of the hindrance of disliking and saying 'disliking', 'disliking', we spin a repetitive story about the person from recycling those angry thoughts. This only makes things worse. Imagine we have to watch a horror movie like Annabelle again and again. Not Annabelle 1, then Annabelle 2, 3, 4 and 5 but just the same Annabelle 1 again and again. For me, I would have passed out.

Most importantly, we need to know that these five things are main factors that stop us from being happy. They are very bad for our practice of mindfulness and happiness. Even if we want to become successful in our life, these five things appear from time to time to stop us. Although they are so bad, but to get rid of them we cannot hate them or chase them away because hating is simply encouraging the hindrance of disliking. The correct way to deal with them is to be mindful of them, to see them clearly, to understand them or even to befriend them. They stop us from progressing, but they are also our greatest teachers. So, pay attention to them!

Exercise 14: identifying hindrances

- Sit comfortably and practice mindful breathing
- If we are distracted, just notice what is the hindrance
- If it is liking, just say 'liking', 'liking'
- If it is disliking, just say 'disliking', 'disliking'
- If it is drowsiness, just say 'drowsiness', 'drowsiness'
- If it is restlessness, just say 'restlessness', 'restlessness'
- If it is doubting, just say 'doubting', 'doubting'
- Observe the arising and the fading away of these hindrances
- When hindrances are absent, return attention to the breath

My grandparents' grocery stall and mindfulness

My grandparents ran a grocery stall at the old Gopeng bus station. As a good grandson, sometimes I helped to sort sweets, candies and snacks of different types, and put them into small packets. Those packets were sealed airtight with candle flame, and sold. Similarly, in mindfulness of thoughts, we sort the different types of thoughts, put them into categories, seal them airtight with the flame of insight, and let them go.

Although mind and thoughts are linked and inseparable, it is useful to separate them initially for the sake of practice. It is good to understand that when we are practicing mindfulness of mind we are paying attention to the overall mental states; and when we are practicing mindfulness of thoughts we are focusing on the individual thoughts and thoughts processes. When we say 'angry', 'angry', we are practicing mindfulness of mind, we are observing the mind as a whole; when we say 'anger', 'anger', we are practicing mindfulness of thoughts. This separation sounds arbitrary but it helps to develop our attention systematically.

The waterfall of thoughts

When we begin to observe our thoughts, we may notice that our thoughts rush and roar like a steep waterfall. But as we continue to observe, they will become a gorge, then a great river flowing down mountains through valleys or along plains, towards the sea. At the end, the mind becomes calm and still like the deep ocean, ruffled by only occasional flickering of thoughts.

Satipatthana Sutta: And how does he in regard to thoughts abide observing thoughts? Here in regard to thoughts he abides observing thoughts in terms of the five hindrances. And how does he in regard to thoughts abide observing thoughts in terms of the five hindrances? If liking [disliking, drowsiness, restlessness, doubt] is present in him, he knows 'There is liking [etc.] in me'; if liking [etc.] is not present in him, he knows 'There is no liking [etc.] in me'; and he knows how unarisen liking [etc.] can arise, how arisen liking [etc.] can be removed, and how a future arising of the removed liking [etc.] can be prevented.

Therefore, the first stage of practicing mindfulness of hindrances requires us to simply observe the presence and the absence of the hindrances in our mind. The second stage is to observe the actual processes of the arising and the fading away of hindrances, looking at the factors that trigger the arising, factors that remove the hindrances, and factors that prevent the future arising of the hindrances.

The point is we can practice mindfulness of the hindrances during any of our mindfulness exercises, such as mindfulness of breathing, postures, activities, body parts, body compositions or decompositions, feelings or mind. But the only difference is the object of attention now is the distraction! We can also practice mindfulness of hindrances when we are doing our work to see what are the thoughts or obstacles that stop us from finishing our job. Meet these hindrances like how we meet our teachers. Greet them. Pay respect to them. Hey! 'Restlessness' Hey! 'Disliking' Observe them. Let them come and go. But don't talk to them. They will tell us what we are still holding on. They will tell us why our practice of mindfulness is not progressing. But don't talk to them or they will stay forever. Just listen to them what they are trying to say. Just learn from them. That is mindfulness of hindrances.

Recycling and mindfulness

Before throwing anything, we need to separate them into plastic, paper and cans. For unwholesome thoughts, we separate them into 'I want', 'I don't want' and 'I don't care' before we throw them into the recycling bins of greed, anger and ignorance. Later, we can then convert them into non-greed (contentment, gratitude and generosity), non-anger (patience, love and compassion) and non-ignorance (understanding, caring and mindfulness).

Mindfulness of the five aggregates (*khandha*)

The five aggregates are the five components that come together to give us our sense of self. They are the body, feelings, perceptions, thoughts and consciousness. When we ask ourselves who we are, we often think we are so and so. But the actual reality is we are the combination of a body and a mind. The mind is divided further into feelings, perceptions, thoughts and consciousness. Feelings here refer to the raw quality of pleasantness, unpleasantness and neutrality. Perceptions are what the mind does to pick up the important characteristics of experiences. Then we have all the thoughts that come up in our mind, wholesome, unwholesome or variable; and lastly consciousness that simply knows. These five aggregates that come together, are who we are. These five are components that give us our sense of self.

So, who am I? Or to be more precise, what am I? I am the five aggregates. These five aggregates are the basis of five types of self-cherishing thoughts, which are 'my body', 'my feelings', 'my perceptions', 'my thoughts' and 'my consciousness'. And this 'I', 'me' or 'mine' actually causes a lot of problems in our life, such as I am stressed, I am sad, I am anxious, I am scared, I like this, I like that, I want this, I want that, I don't want this, I don't want that. The list can be very long. But we must see for ourselves that all problems stem from this 'I'. No I. No problem. When the sense of I is not present, not there, the body, feelings, perceptions, thoughts and consciousness remain. It is just that we no longer identify with it so much. Then, all the problems that arise from such identification disappear. No I, no problem.

So, in mindfulness of the aggregates we pay attention to the different components that make up our sense of self. We observe how we identify with the aggregates as being 'I' or 'mine'. As we watch the arising and fading away of these five aggregates, we may be able to see that this thing we called 'I', that we cling to for our whole life, is just a mere collection of subjective experiences of the body, feelings, perceptions, thoughts and consciousness. As a result of this understanding, instead of saying 'I am depressed', we say 'depression', 'depression'. Instead of saying 'I am in pain', we say 'pain', 'pain'. Understanding this impersonal nature of our experiences, we then won't take things so personally.

Among all the thoughts of the fourth aggregate, intention is being singled out as one of the most important thoughts. Intention is concerned with the actualization of a goal. It is the chief of our mind that leads the other thoughts to achieve a purpose. Intention is ethically neutral but the wholesomeness or unwholesomeness of an action is determined by the motivation associated with the intention.

In mindfulness of aggregates we observe the subjective experiences of our body, our feelings, our perceptions, our thoughts and our consciousness, closely. We observe the arising and fading away of these subjective experiences. We observe our identification with each component and we observe the problems that come from this identification.

When we observe thoughts, we pay particular attention to the chief of our mind, the intention. We observe the arising of our intentions during our breathing, our postures, and our activities. We observe our intentions before, during and after breathing in; before, during and after breathing out. We observe them before, during and after we adopt a posture. And we observe them before, during and after we perform an activity. We pay attention to the stream of intentions that begins, maintains and stops our every breath, posture and activity. Is each of our intentions wholesome or unwholesome? We observe our intentions closely.

Then we try to find the 'I' in our intentions. We try to locate it. Is there an independent entity called 'I' that controls all these intentions? Or are these intentions dependent on multiple other factors such as the body, feelings, perceptions, thoughts, emotions and consciousness? The intention is often a hideout for our sense of 'I'. Search thoroughly for this 'I'!

This 'I' or sense of self is not necessary in our pursuit of happiness. Not only it is not necessary but it actually blocks our happiness. All our unwholesome thoughts and **hindrances** arise from our ego or selfishness. All our unwholesome speeches and actions arise from our ego too. Speak and act with a selfish mind and stress and suffering will follow us. Speak and act with a selfless mind and happiness will follow us. When we start to stop taking our 'self' personally, and start to consider 'others' in the picture, we will notice ourselves suffering less and less, and getting happier and happier.

The evolution of the material 'Me' with mindfulness practice

First, we become mindful materialists, then mindful minimalists and minimal-'me'-lists. Finally, the 'me' disappears and what is left is purely mindful minimalism.

Exercise 15: observing the five aggregates

- As we practice the second stage of mindfulness of hindrances in exercise 14, we observe the arising and falling of hindrances
- We may realize that the reason of the arising of hindrances is because of our sense of self
- Our sense of self wants to gratify ourselves with pleasure
- Our sense of self wants to avoid pain and suffering
- Observe this sense of self throughout the day
- How strong is our sense of self?
- At which time of the day is it strongest?
- In what roles and situations is it strongest?

- How does it feel when it is strongest?
- How does the body feel?
- How does it affect others?
- Ask ourselves who am I during that time?
- Am I the body?
- Am I the stream of changing feelings?
- Am I the perceptions?
- Am I the thoughts, ideas, views, beliefs and hopes?
- Am I the consciousness?
- Who am I?
- Notice which aggregate are we identifying with most
- Notice which aggregate are we clinging to most strongly
- Which one can we easily let go?
- Observe when is this sense of self weakest or absent in the day
- How does it feel when it is weakest or absent?
- How does the body feel?
- How does it affect others?
- Then, imagine there is no self
- Let all experience be like a movie without clinging to any of the aggregates or taking it personally
- How does it feel?
- How does the body feel?
- How does it affect others?
- Can we function well without our sense of self?
- Can we see that our sense of self is created by our identification with the five aggregates?
- Can we realize that the less we cling to our sense of self, the freer and happier we will be?

Satipatthana Sutta: Again, in regard to thoughts he abides observing thoughts in terms of the five aggregates of clinging. And how does he in regard to thoughts abide observing thoughts in terms of the five aggregates of clinging. Here he knows, 'Such is the body, such its arising, such its falling; such is feeling, such its arising, such its falling; such is perception, such its arising, such its falling; such is thought, such its arising, such its falling; such is consciousness, such its arising, such its falling.'

Mindfulness of the six sense-spheres (*ayatana*)

The six sense-spheres can be internal or external. The six internal sense-spheres refer to the six sense bases, namely eyes, ears, nose, tongue, body and mind. The external sense-spheres refer to their respective sense objects, namely forms, sounds, odors, tastes, bodily sensations and thoughts. While mindfulness of aggregates enables us to realize the contribution of the sense of self that arises from the identification with the five aggregates to our daily problems, mindfulness of the six sense-spheres allows us to see the problems that arise from our relationship between ourselves and the outer world.

The roof and mindfulness

Built in the 18th century, my grandparents' shophouse was not water-proof. During heavy rainstorm, we had to use pots and containers of all kinds to collect water dripping from the leaky roof. That was how I created music without any inspiration from Kitaro. The music was nice but the roof might collapse if we didn't repair it. In a similar sense, to repair our psychological well-being, we need to put six security guards of mindfulness at the six sense-spheres to prevent leaking in of negativities of all sorts.

Satipatthana Sutta: In regard to thoughts, one abides observing thoughts in terms of the six internal and external sense-spheres. And how does one abide observing thoughts in terms of the six internal and external sense-spheres? Here, one knows the eyes [etc.], one knows forms [etc.], and one knows the fetter that arises dependent on both, and one also knows how an unarisen fetter can arise, how an arisen fetter can be removed, and how a future arising of the removed fetter can be prevented.

Fetter is a chain used to restrain a prisoner. It is used here to describe how the six sense-spheres, chain us like a prisoner, not allowing us to be free. Examples of fetters include greed, anger, ignorance, arrogance, self-centeredness, jealousy, restlessness, doubt, attachment to rites and rituals and wrong views. These are basically unwholesome or negative thoughts that bind us in our day-to-day life; that make us anxious, fearful, depressed, restless or stressed; that stop us from being free. We may not need to follow the list, but every time we feel we are not free, bound by problems, disturbing thoughts or overwhelming emotions, we can practice mindfulness of the fetters that arise through the six sense-spheres.

Exercise 16: identifying fetters or unwholesome thoughts

- Make ourselves comfortable
- Relax our body
- Take two deep breaths
- Then breathe naturally
- Pay attention to our six sense-spheres
- Be aware of our eyes and our vision
- Be aware of the fetters that arise from this sense-sphere
- Like seeing people we like and people we don't like
- Be aware of our ears and our hearing
- Be aware of the fetters that arise from this sense-sphere
- Like hearing comments we like and comments we don't like
- Be aware of our nose and our smelling
- Be aware of the fetters that arise from this sense-sphere
- Like smelling odor we like and odor we don't like
- Be aware of our tongue and our tasting
- Be aware of the fetters that arise from this sense-sphere

- Like tasting food we like and tasting food we don't like
- Be aware of our body and our feeling
- Be aware of the fetters that arise from this sense-sphere
- Like feeling pleasure and pain
- Be aware of our mind and our thoughts
- Be aware of the fetters that arise from this sense-sphere
- Like thinking about things we like or things we don't like
- Mental noting: fetters-fetters or *samyojana-samyojana*
- Observe how an unarisen fetter can arise
- Observe how an arisen fetter can be removed
- Observe how a removed fetter can be prevented from arising
- Cultivate mindfulness at the six sense-spheres
- Let mindfulness be our guardian of the sense doors
- Let mindfulness be our protector of the mind
- Protecting us from all the fetters or negative thoughts

In mindfulness of hindrances, we focus on the five categories of unwholesome thoughts that block our mindfulness practice. In mindfulness of aggregates, we focus on the five types of self-cherishing thoughts that serve as a basis for the arising of unwholesome thoughts. In mindfulness of sense-spheres, we train in observing the external and internal sources of stressful thoughts. These three practices bring us face-to-face with our stress factors from a gross level to subtler levels. When we are familiar with recognizing these thoughts that block psychological freedom and encourage cognitive inflexibility, we remove them.

Mindfulness of the seven awakening factors (*bojjhanga*)

Bojjhanga means awakening factors or factors that wake us up. It wakes us up from our automatic pilot of our day-to-day routines. It is like making us feeling alive again instead of roaming the streets like zombies with our cell-phones. But of course we can scroll our cell-phones mindfully too. It wakes us up from the vicious cycles of stress and suffering. It wakes us up from our sleep and unconsciousness of what is happening around us and what is happening inside our mind. Just like the river flows towards the ocean, the seven awakening factors flow towards the complete cessation of stress.

They are seven awakening factors. We can call them stress-cessation factors. The first is the chief awakening factors that lead all the other 6 factors – mindfulness (sati). After talking about mindfulness from the beginning until now I am sure we are aware of the importance of mindfulness as a chief factor in stress cessation. In order for mindfulness to become an awakening factor, it has to be strong and focused, established in the four foundations, with the four mental qualities and four refrains.

In fact, when mindfulness is stable and continuous, all the other factors arise automatically. That means when we are practicing mindfulness correctly, the seven awakening factors are being practiced too. The next three factors are literally awakening factors because they give us energy when our mind is in a low energy state, like when we are drowsy, tired, bored or lazy. These three factors are introspection, diligence, and joy. They are particularly useful to overcome the hindrance of drowsiness.

Introspection (vicaya) here refers to using mindfulness to look inside our mind. We investigate our body, our feelings, our perceptions, our thoughts and our consciousness. We apply our skills of mindfulness on every aspects of our life and activities of daily living. We observe our wholesome and unwholesome thoughts in every activity. We practice mindfulness to cultivate wholesome mental states and abandon unwholesome mental states in all situations.

Next, we have diligence (*viriya*). Diligence is the skillful balance of effort in practicing mindfulness. If we are too lazy to practice, diligence gives us energy to continue practice. If we are overenthusiastic and obsessed in practicing, diligence reminds us to slow down and be kind to ourselves. *Viriya* is similar to *atapi*. Both are willpower.

Then we have joy (*piti*). If we do not have joy while we are practicing mindfulness, we will have stopped practicing in the very beginning. The correct practice of mindfulness always has an element of joy. If we are sweeping the floor mindfully, joy will arise. If we are driving mindfully in a traffic jam, joy will arise. If we are queueing mindfully at McDonald, joy will arise. Joy is a pleasant feeling not associated with desire. It is an unworldly pleasant feeling that is unpolluted by unwholesome thoughts, if we still remember the chapter on mindfulness of feelings.

The last three factors are useful to overcome the hindrance of restlessness. These three factors are tranquility, concentration and equanimity. When we are mindful enough, joy will arise. When joy arises, tranquility (*passaddhi*) will follow. Tranquility means the body is relaxed and the mind is calm. We will feel very comfortable and at ease. As we feel at ease, the mind will develop concentration (*samadhi*). The mind will become clearer; hindrances will fade to the background. As our concentration deepens, our mind will be very focused, like a laser beam. We can apply this laser beam to see our mind and thoughts clearly.

The practice and development of concentration leads to equanimity when the hindrances are secluded from the mind. Equanimity (*upekkha*) is a state of psychological stability and composure which is unaffected by unwholesome thoughts and emotions. When equanimity is present, we will not be disturbed by the eight vicissitudes of life, namely loss and gain; fame and shame; praise and blame; pleasure and pain.

Again there are two stages in the practice of mindfulness of awakening factors. The first stage is to know the presence and absence of awakening factors. The second stage is to know the conditions that lead to the arising of the awakening factors if they are absent; and the conditions that lead to further development and perfection if they are present.

Satipatthana Sutta: Here, if the mindfulness awakening factor [etc.] is present in him, he knows 'There is mindfulness awakening factor [etc.] in me'; if the mindfulness awakening factor [etc.] is not present in him, he knows 'There is no mindfulness awakening factor [etc.] in me'; he knows how the unarisen mindfulness awakening factor [etc.] can arise, and how the arisen mindfulness awakening factor [etc.] can be perfected by development.

Exercise 17: knowing the presence/absence of awakening factors

- Practice mindfulness of breathing
- Sit upright
- Make ourselves comfortable
- Relax our body
- Rest our attention on our breathing
- Then observe whether mindfulness is present or not
- If mindfulness is present, we know there is mindfulness
- If mindfulness is absent, we know there is no mindfulness
- Observe the arising and falling of mindfulness
- Recognize factors that condition the arising of mindfulness
- And factors that condition the perfection of mindfulness
- Mental noting: *sati-sati-sati*
- Practice mindfulness to investigate the nature of our body, our feelings, our mind and our thoughts
- Investigate the nature of arising and falling of each experience
- Investigate the conditioning of the arising and falling
- If introspection is present, we know there is introspection
- If introspection is absent, we know there is no introspection

- Observe the arising and falling of introspection
- Recognize factors that condition the arising of introspection
- And factors that condition the perfection of introspection
- Mental noting: *vicaya-vicaya-vicaya*
- Make effort to be mindful when mindfulness is weak or absent
- Reduce effort when we notice we are striving too hard
- Be aware of the right amount of effort to be mindful
- If diligence is present, we know there is diligence
- If diligence is absent, we know there is no diligence
- Observe the arising and falling of diligence
- Recognize factors that condition the arising of diligence
- And factors that condition the perfection of diligence
- Mental noting: *viriya-viriya-viriya*
- With mindfulness, investigation and effort, joy will arise
- Observe the presence and absence of this joy of mindfulness
- If joy is present, we know there is joy
- If joy is absent, we know there is no joy
- Observe the arising and falling of joy
- Recognize factors that condition the arising of joy
- And factors that condition the perfection of joy
- Mental noting: *piti-piti-piti*
- When we are joyful, tranquility will arise
- Observe the presence and absence of tranquility
- If tranquility is present, we know there is tranquility
- The body is relaxed and the mind is calm
- We remain calm with the eight vicissitudes in life
- Pleasure and pain
- Loss and gain
- Praise and blame
- Fame and shame
- If tranquility is absent, we know there is no tranquility
- The body is tense and the mind is restless
- Observe the arising and falling of tranquility
- Recognize factors that condition the arising of tranquility
- And factors that condition the perfection of tranquility

- Mental noting: *passaddhi-passaddhi-passaddhi*
- When our mind is calm, concentration will arise
- Observe the presence and absence of concentration
- If concentration is present, we know there is concentration
- We have overcome the five hindrances
- If concentration is absent, we know there is no concentration
- Observe the arising and falling of concentration
- Recognize factors that condition the arising of concentration
- And factors that condition the perfection of concentration
- Mental noting: *samadhi-samadhi-samadhi*
- When our mind is concentrated, equanimity will arise
- Observe the presence and absence of equanimity
- If equanimity is present, we know there is equanimity
- We are unaffected by hindrances or unwholesome thoughts
- If equanimity is absent, we know there is no equanimity
- Observe the arising and falling of equanimity
- Recognize factors that condition the arising of equanimity
- And factors that condition the perfection of equanimity
- Mental noting: *upekkha-upekkha-upekkha*

Mindfulness of the four noble truths (*sacca*)

The four noble truths referred to suffering (*dukkha*), causes of suffering (*samudaya*), cessation of suffering (*nirodha*) and the paths leading to the cessation of suffering (*magga*). Mindfulness of the four noble truths involves the integration of all the previous exercises into our day-to-day life.

Mindfulness of the body begins with mindful breathing as an essential starting point in anchoring our attention, followed by the four postures, daily activities, body parts, body compositions and decompositions. Then it progresses from these immediately accessible physical experiences to mindfulness of feelings, which is more refined and subtle.

Mindfulness of feelings begins from observing the affective qualities of pleasure, pain and neutral sensations to observing the ethical qualities of worldly and unworldly feelings. The latter prepares us for mindfulness of mind that begins with observing the wholesomeness and unwholesomeness of our mind, followed by observing the different meditative states of a mindful mind.

The awareness of the different meditative states of a mindful mind prepares us to investigate the various thoughts that hinder progress – mindfulness of the five hindrances, followed by subtler unwholesome thoughts of our sense of self – mindfulness of the five aggregates, and unwholesome thoughts that bind us to the stress and hassles of our daily life – mindfulness of the fetters.

Next, we proceed with the practice of mindfulness of the seven awakening factors. These psychological factors are factors that are anti-hindrances, anti-ego, and anti-fetters. Practicing these psychological factors lead us naturally to the complete cessation of stress and suffering in life.

Finally, we practice mindfulness of the four noble truths, in which the first two are concerned with the observing of the arising of stress and suffering in life due to the five hindrances, the five aggregates and the fetters. The latter two noble truths are concerned with the observing of the cessation of stress and suffering in life due to the unfolding of the awakening factors.

Therefore, mindfulness of the four noble truths involves integrating everything that we have learnt from the *satipatthana* into every activities of our daily life, especially in our thoughts, speeches and actions. First noble truth: In the truth of suffering, it was explained that suffering is not inherent in the nature of our mind. It exists only in the way the ordinary mind experiences it. It arises when we are not able to accept changes, such as birth, aging, sickness and death. It also arises when we cannot accept situations such as separating from who we love, not getting what we want, getting what we don't want and clinging to our negative experiences.

Second noble truth: The three root causes of our suffering are thoughts of attachment, aversion and delusion. Attachment is the craving of things we like. Aversion is the hating of things we dislike. Delusion means not being mindful, not seeing things as they are, and being ignorant to the reality. It includes the four mistaken beliefs that the body is beautiful (reality: the body is just as it is, it is our biased judgment that makes it beautiful, or not), that enduring happiness is achieved through enjoying pleasure and avoiding pain (reality: pleasure is transient, pain is inevitable in life), that things are permanent (reality: things change), that our self is an independent entity (reality: the self is conditioned by the five aggregates, even the intention is conditioned; when any of the aggregate is absent, the sense of self disappears).

Each foundation of mindfulness is supposed to address one of the four mistaken beliefs. Mindfulness of the body allows us to observe the body as it is, and helps us to see the impurities inside our body. Mindfulness of feelings allows us to recognize that our habitual reactions to pleasure and pain are not a good solution to happiness. Mindfulness of mind allows us to see the impermanent nature of our mind. Mindfulness of thoughts helps us to see the conditioned nature of our self, that we are conditioned by the body, feelings, perceptions, thoughts and consciousness. In the absence of any of these components, the sense of self will lose its clinging.

The third truth speaks about the inherent nature of our mind which is free from all negative thoughts. It is a radical freedom that is independent of favourable or unfavourable conditions. The fourth truth speaks about the eight strategies leading to this freedom of mind, namely right understanding, right intention, right speech, right action, right livelihood, right effort, right mindfulness and right concentration.

Right intention, speech, action and livelihood are training in morality. Right effort, mindfulness and concentration are training in calming the mind and looking inside to familiarize ourselves with our mind. Right understanding is the insight that follows from the training in morality and familiarization with our mind.

As we practice mindfulness of the body, we calm down our body. As we practice mindfulness of feelings, we recognize our ingrained habitual reactions to feelings. Practicing mindfulness of mind, we recognize the wholesomeness and unwholesomeness of different mental states. Practicing mindfulness of thoughts, we recognize different types of thoughts that block psychological freedom, followed by different types of thoughts that lead to psychological freedom.

The four noble truths summarize all the instructions and strategies in achieving lasting happiness. Mindfulness of the four noble truths requires us to observe our mind whenever we are suffering in life; to observe the factors leading to those suffering; to observe our mind when we are free from suffering, and to observe the factors leading to the freedom from suffering.

Exercise 18: observing the four noble truths in our daily life

- Make a conscious effort to bring mindfulness to our whole day
- Breathing in, we know we are breathing in
- Breathing out, we know we are breathing out
- Use mindful breathing as an anchor in practicing mindfulness
- Pick a few things as gentle reminders of mindfulness
- We may use mindfulness bell as reminder of mindful breathing
- We may use traffic light as reminder of mindful driving

- We may use long corridor as reminder of mindful walking
- We may use sink water as reminder of mindful hand washing
- We may use someone's eyes as reminder of mindful presence
- Be mindful of suffering throughout the day
- When suffering is present, we acknowledge its presence
- We do not ignore, suppress or blame on situations or others
- We do not resist the very idea of our own suffering
- Observe the actual experience of suffering as it really is
- Observe the actual experience without creating any stories
- Observe suffering to fully understand it
- Then, integrate this full understanding into our life
- This is mindfulness of the first noble truth
- Acknowledging suffering
- Knowing suffering as it is
- Integrating this knowledge into our life
- Be mindful of the internal causes of suffering
- Observe the arising of suffering from the three root causes
- Is our suffering due to our craving of something pleasant?
- Is our suffering due to our hating of something unpleasant?
- Is our suffering due to our sense of self?
- Abandon these causes of suffering
- Then, integrate this knowledge into our life
- This is mindfulness of the second noble truth
- Seeing the causes of suffering
- Abandoning the causes of suffering
- Integrating this knowledge into our life
- Be mindful of freedom from suffering throughout the day
- When suffering ceases, we feel fresh, calm and relaxed
- We are free from craving, hating and ignoring
- Experience this freedom mindfully
- Free from the three unwholesome mental states
- Free from the five hindrances
- Free from clinging to the five aggregates
- Free from all fetters and unwholesome thoughts
- Then, let this freedom manifests throughout our life

- Knowing that nothing lasts
- Knowing that it is nothing personal
- This is mindfulness of the third noble truth
- Experiencing the freedom from suffering
- Fully understanding the freedom from suffering as it is
- Manifesting this freedom from suffering throughout life
- Be mindful of the eight strategies leading to suffering cessation
- Be mindful of how right understanding leads to freedom
- Understanding suffering
- Understanding the causes of suffering
- Understanding the cessation of suffering
- Understanding the eight strategies of suffering cessation
- Be mindful of how right intention leads to freedom
- Intention to do no harm
- Intention to do good
- Intention to purify our mind
- Be mindful of how right speech leads to freedom
- Speaking truthfully
- Speaking respectfully
- Speaking gently
- Speaking usefully
- Speaking timely
- Be mindful of how right action leads to freedom
- Doing no harm
- Not taking what is not given
- Not involving in inappropriate sex
- Not lying
- Not consuming unhealthy food and beverage
- Be mindful of how right livelihood leads to freedom
- Choosing an ethical profession
- Working with love and compassion
- Be mindful of how right effort leads to freedom
- Effort in preventing arising of unwholesome mental states
- Effort in abandoning arisen unwholesome mental states
- Effort in cultivating arising of wholesome mental states

- Effort in sustaining arisen wholesome mental states
- Be mindful of how right mindfulness leads to freedom
- Mindfulness of the impurities of the body
- Mindfulness of the unsatisfactory nature of feelings
- Mindfulness of the arising and falling of mental states
- Mindfulness of the conditionality of thoughts
- Be mindful of how right concentration leads to freedom
- Concentration to remain calm
- Concentration to see things clearly as they are
- Practice and experience the eight strategies in our life
- Then, integrate the practice into every aspect of our life
- Observe the arising of the seven awakening factors from practicing the eight strategies of suffering cessation
- This is mindfulness of the fourth noble truth
- Reflecting on the eight strategies in suffering cessation
- Practicing and directly experiencing the eight strategies
- Integrating the strategies into every aspect of our life

Satipatthana Sutta: Here one knows as it really is, 'this is suffering'; one knows as it really is, 'this is the arising of suffering'; one knows as it really is, 'this is the cessation of suffering'; one knows as it really is, 'this is the way leading to the cessation of suffering.' In this way, in regard to thoughts we abide observing our own thoughts, the thoughts of others, and both, in terms of the five hindrances of practice, the five aggregates of sense of self, the fetters from the six sense-spheres, the seven awakening factors and the four noble truths. We observe the arising of these thoughts, the passing away of these thoughts, and both. We practice mindfulness of these thoughts to the extent necessary for bare knowledge and continuous mindfulness. And we abide independently not clinging to anything in the world.

And here, I have tried my very best to introduce you to what mindfulness is from the original source – the *Satipatthana Sutta*. The practice is now all up to you. Happy practice!

True love and mindfulness

When my two daughters were born, I became the happiest person in the world. They taught me what true love is, i.e. to share our happiness unconditionally. Just as true love is incomplete without mindfulness; mindfulness is incomplete without love. If we want to be happy, we can practice mindfulness with love; if we want others to be happy, we have to love others mindfully.

Conclusion

Satipatthana Sutta: If anyone should develop these four *satipatthanas* in such a way for seven years, one of the two results could be expected for him: either complete cessation of stress here and now, or, if there is a trace of clinging left, irreversible partial cessation of stress. Let alone seven years... six years... five years... four years... three years... two years... one year... seven months... six months... five months... four months... three months... two months... one month... half a month... if anyone should develop these four *satipatthanas* in such a way for seven days, one of the two results could be expected for him: either complete cessation of stress here and now, or, if there is a trace of clinging left, irreversible partial cessation of stress.

So it was with reference to this that it was said: This is the direct path for the purification of our mind, for the overcoming of sorrow and lamentation, for the relief of physical and mental suffering, for seeing things as they are, and for the experiencing of the complete cessation of stress.

Mindfulness-Based Supportive Therapy (MBST)

Introduction

Mindfulness-based supportive therapy is a love story. The first part of the story is about suffering. When I first joined University of Malaya in 2008, I was strongly encouraged to do research and write scientific papers. In my mind I wanted to do something that I have strong passion in it. So I chose the four noble truths. I wanted to know more about suffering, causes of suffering, cessation of suffering and the causes of cessation of suffering in the end-of-life setting.

To understand suffering I need to understand the subjective experiences of patients. So instead of doing quantitative research like most of my colleagues, I decided to start with qualitative methods first. During that time I have no idea how to conduct qualitative research. I was being introduced to a nursing lecturer with experience in qualitative research. She asked me which method I wanted to use. And she gave me a list of methods. I had no idea what the different methods meant so I went to one of my favourite bookshops – Kinokuniya at Kuala Lumpur Convention Center (KLCC). And I bought some books on research, including a book called Qualitative Psychology by Jonathan Smith.

In 2012, I published my first paper on the experiences of suffering of palliative care patients. That paper was the hardest to publish because it was rejected multiple times. But I am thankful to all the reviewers who commented on that paper because those comments help me to improve.

After the first paper on suffering, I moved on to publish the experiences of suffering of palliative care family caregivers, the experiences of stress of palliative care providers, suffering caused by healthcare providers, measuring suffering in palliative care with the suffering pictogram, the experiences of well-being of palliative care patients, etc., etc., all about suffering and cessation of suffering because Bruce Lee said it is better to practice one kick 10,000 times rather than 10,000 different types of kicks.

The second part of the story is about mindfulness. Back in 1998, I did my elective posting at Hualien Tzu Chi Hospital. Beside the hospital canteen, I met Master Cheng Yen, the founder of the Tzu Chi Foundation. She said to me and my friends, "You are all from Malaysia. One day you will all become great doctors. Use your heart." But I didn't understand the exact meaning of 'use your heart'.

Fast forward to 2008, you can imagine those images in your mind now suddenly flash rapidly in front of you like when you are watching a movie and someone presses the fast forward button... I started to have more time for myself after coming back from Singapore where I did my fellowship in palliative care. I began to read more books on mindfulness. My favourite one is Present Moment Wonderful Moment by the Vietnamese Master Thich Nhat Hanh. The book contains many mindfulness verses called *gathas* that I can use to integrate mindfulness into my day-to-day life. It is a little bit like what everyone called 'mindful living'.

I also started to meditate after reading The Joy of Living by Yongey Mingyur Rinpoche. He is a happy Tibetan monk. Then I noticed after months of meditation practices, my stress level dropped to zero. I still experience stress once in a while but it disappears quickly once I am aware of it and stop sustaining it. I am able to regulate my stress and emotions much better.

Then, I realized that 'use your heart' is exactly the same as mindfulness, exactly the same! Can you imagine? Master Cheng Yen planted the seeds of mindfulness in me during the brief encounter. The seeds grew only after more than a decade! Now I am appreciating its flower and enjoying its fruit. Mindfulness, it really has become an indispensable asset for me. Mindfulness protects me from being overwhelmed by the intense emotions in palliative care. It gives me a *psychological holiday*. This is why I never take leave due to exhaustion reasons. But I do take leave during Chinese New Year and during time when I need to take care of my children, not forgetting my wonderful carefree sabbatical leave every three years!

Then I started to notice this mindfulness of breathing that I practiced during sitting meditation has seeped into my life, including my work. When I saw patients, they could be telling me all of their distress and frustration, I could feel them but I wasn't affected by them. My mindfulness of breathing was still with me. It was then I decided to marry my work on suffering with my passion in mindfulness. To be honest, mindfulness, is not only my passion, it is also my wife, my life, my religion. Don't worry my wife won't be reading this book. She is too busy. And I published my first mindfulness paper on Mindfulness-Based Supportive Therapy (MBST), a book on mindfulness called The Little Handbook of Mini-Mindfulness Meditation (MMM) because I like to eat M&M chocolate, and a few other mindfulness papers.

The conceptualization of MBST was done in three phases. First, a theory of suffering was formulated by merging the two models of suffering in palliative care from my previous studies. Open-ended questions from the first two studies of suffering were formulated to assess suffering. Types of suffering from the two studies were used as a guide in the diagnosis of suffering.

Second, the framework of MBST was formed from matching the themes of healthcare-related suffering to potential solutions, namely presence, listening, empathy, compassion and boundary issues. Third, principles of mindfulness were incorporated into the framework to form MBST.

MBST is specifically designed for healthcare providers to practice during their encounter with palliative care patients and family caregivers. It allows healthcare providers to continue their practice of mindfulness during patient care. The benefits include (1) Flexibility – there is no restriction in time, number of sessions; it can be delivered by any healthcare providers to patients, family members or both; it can be terminated at any time; and it can be a bridge to other psychotherapies, (2) Reciprocity – it may alleviate suffering of patients and family members; at the very least, it may reduce stress of healthcare providers, (3) Simultaneity – it allows healthcare providers to practice mindfulness during work, i.e. no change in working schedule.

Satipatthana Sutta: In regard to the body [feelings, mind and thoughts], one abides observing the body internally, **EXTERNALLY** and both. One abides observing the nature of arising in the body [feelings, mind and thoughts], the nature of disappearing and both. Mindfulness that 'there is a body' [feelings, mind and thoughts] is established to the extent necessary for bare knowledge and continuous mindfulness. And one abides independently, not clinging to anything in the world.

If we still remember, the above paragraph is the refrain of *Satipatthana Sutta*. It appears 13 different times after each mindfulness exercise, showing how important it is. The word externally means observing the body, feelings, mind and thoughts of another person. The whole practice of MBST is about the practice of observing internally, **EXTERNALLY** and both.

It is important to know that the *satipatthanas* do prepare us for the next stage of practice, i.e. practicing mindfulness when we are with others. If we are mindful enough, we may be able to spread some mindfulness to others. At the very least, we have the advantage to continue our practice even when we are with others. So let us practice MBST together, and be joyfully together. This is going to be my motto for the rest of my working life: practice MBST together, be joyfully together!!

Mindful Presence

Introduction

The most important gift we can offer for our patients and their family members is our presence. Presence itself is therapeutic in its own sense. According to Hines, presence is a mode of being available in a situation with the wholeness of one's unique individual being. That means when we are present, we are giving the whole of ourselves to the person we are with, the WHOLE of ourselves. We are completely there for them at that moment in time.

Three types of presence have been described in the literature by Stiles in 1997. First is physical presence, means being there. This is a body-to-body type of presence. The barriers for physical presence are busyness, rushing all the time and excessively task-orientated. If we are not there physically, we cannot talk about presence. Of course I can ask my children to hug my bolster when I go oversea. I can ask them to treat my bolster as me. But it is not the same. My bolster is a bolster. It cannot replace me.

Second is psychological presence, means being with and connecting with patients with empathy. This is a mind-to-mind contact. The barrier for psychological presence is the lack of concern. It is like yes we are at home with our family but we are completely engrossed in doing our own things. I am reading my books. My wife is watching ASTRO without blinking. My children are playing their I-pads. That is not presence too. We can do our own things but we have to recognize the presence of each other, not just 'be there', but also 'be with'.

Third is a special form of presence. It is a spiritual presence or a healing presence. It means 'being', 'to be', 'just be', with inner quietude and mindfulness. This is a soul-to-soul contact. Barriers are cognitive, emotional or behavioural reactivity, the urge to do something, and 'doing'. For spiritual presence, we empty our mind from all our reactivity and create a safe space for the person to be with us. This can be achieved by practicing mindful presence.

The dying baby

I remember seeing a dying baby during one of my home visits. He lied motionlessly in a cot with a feeding tube placed through his nose into his stomach. He was affected by excessive accumulation of fluid in the brain, a condition called hydrocephalus that caused his head to look bigger than usual. I couldn't imagine the pain his mother was going through. She looked extremely haggard. She told me she didn't sleep well because she was watching her baby's breathing the whole night, fearing that his breathing might stop anytime if she fell asleep. I was deeply touched by her love. After that, I give the whole of myself to my daughters whenever I am with them, knowing that they will die too one day.

In the practice of mindful presence, first we practice mindful breathing. We observe our in-breath and out-breath. Breathing in, we know we are breathing in. Breathing out, we know we are breathing out. We follow the entire length of our breath. In-in-in. Out-out-out. We feel our whole body and relax our whole body. Then we pay full attention to our own presence and the presence of others. By coming back to our breathing and our body, we can feel more alive, and we can make others feel more alive too. We sustain our attention on this collective presence, just like we are completely there for patients.

In mindful presence, eye contact is very important. We have to train ourselves to be able to maintain good eye contact with patients. Look into patients' eyes. Don't stare at their eyes as if we want to laser their lens or laser them, like the Godzilla laser eyes. Also don't gaze at them as if our eyes are glued to theirs, like when we fall in love with someone, but just relax our gaze. Breathe in. Breathe out. Relax our gaze. Look into their eyes.

Keep part of our attention on our breathing, and part of our attention on their eyes. Relax our eye muscles. Relax and expand our vision from looking into patients' eyes to looking at their faces. Observe his or her facial expression. Then expand our vision further to include the whole body while maintaining our eye contact. Observe his or her breathing, body postures and body movement, the same way when we are practicing mindfulness of the body (*kayanupassana*) in *satipatthana*. The only difference now is we are practicing not only internally, but internally (mindfulness of our own body), externally (mindfulness of the body of others) and both.

And how, do we in regard to the body abide observing the body of a patient? Here, when we see a patient in the hospital, or in the clinic, or during home visit, we establish mindfulness in front of us, mindfully we observe the patient breathing in when patient is breathing in, and mindfully we observe the patient breathing out when patient is breathing out.

When patient is breathing in long, we know patient is breathing in long. When patient is breathing out long, we know patient is breathing out long. When patient is breathing in short, we know patient is breathing in short. When patient is breathing out short, we know patient is breathing out short. In this way, we pay attention to the entire length of patient's breathing.

We observe the eyes, the face and the whole body of patient when patient is breathing. We pay attention to his or her posture. When patient is walking, we know patient is walking; when patient is standing, we know patient is standing; when patient is sitting, we know patient is sitting; when patient is lying down, we know patient is lying down; and we know accordingly what his or her body posture is.

When patient is walking toward us or away from us we are clearly aware; when patient is looking at us or looking away from us we are clearly aware; when patient is flexing or extending his or her limbs we are clearly aware; when patient is removing wrinkles of his or her dress, or carrying his or her tubes and lines we are clearly aware; when patient is eating and drinking we are clearly aware; when patient is walking, standing, sitting, falling asleep, waking up, talking, and keeping silent we are clearly aware. We are clearly aware of the purpose of his or her activity, whether it is wholesome or unwholesome; clearly aware of the appropriateness of the activity; clearly aware of the field of practice of our mindfulness; and clearly aware of the activity as it is without adding our own judgment.

We can keep 50% of our attention on our in and out-breath, and 50% of our attention on patient. And when our mindfulness is stable, we can switch most of our attention to patient, say 90%. Keep at least 10% attention on our breathing so we are still aware of what is happening to ourselves while paying attention to what is happening to patient. I will explain more on this when I talk about mindfulness of boundaries. The percentages we use here are arbitrary figures. They are given to serve as a rough guide as to how we can divide our attention, but not to be followed blindly.

Next, be aware that the body of patients are made of the same constituents as our body, same skin, muscles, bones, and same organs. Be aware that the very body of patients is of the same nature as ours, subjected to the same processes of aging, sickness, death and decomposition. Again the correct attitude is needed in practicing this section, which is to see things as they really are, but not to get attracted to the superficial part of the body or feel disgusted about the internal organs and body fluids.

If we notice we are judging patients, we come back to our breathing gently. If we find ourselves feeling anxious or rushed, we return our attention to our breathing. We practice coming back again and again to our breathing and our presence. We practice to be there completely for patients, not thinking about the past or future, not thinking about lunch or dinner.

When we see a patient or a family caregiver in the hospital, we can practice mindful presence. When we see our colleagues in the office or at the corridor, we can practice mindful presence. We may call this practice: 'mindful presence at the corridor'. This can be very useful especially for those who meet a lot of people at the corridor. I seem to be one of them. They often asked me, "How are you?" at the corridor, but before I could smile or respond to them they already walked past me. So I ended up practicing mindful smiling.

When we are with our family members and friends, we can practice mindful presence. Just sit there and be there for them completely. Look at them properly. Look at their eyes. And see what happens next. Who knows the next day they may buy us a new I-phone or a new pair of shoes. But if they continue to watch television, that is ok. Just be mindful of our own breath and recognize their presence, or practice mindful smiling.

When we meet a stranger on the street we can also practice mindful presence. Even when we are in a crowd, we can practice mindful presence. We see a person. We breathe in and out. We come back to the present moment. We come back to our body. And be present for the person fully. Add a little smile to our presence. Not too much, not too little. Just a little smile, like when we are feeling very calm. If it is too much, we may look weird. If it is too little, we may look very fierce.

In this way, every time we see a person, it becomes an opportunity for us to practice mindfulness. Every person that we meet becomes a support for our practice of mindfulness. In some situations, our presence may not be needed, like when patient is too tired, or when our family member is too engrossed in doing something, or when our friends are too busy. Then, we can just practice mindful breathing. Don't be overenthusiastic!

Instructions for mindful presence

- Start with a wholesome intention to practice mindful presence
- Sit down at the same eye level with a patient
- Keep a comfortable distance
- Maintain an open posture
- Keep our arms and legs uncrossed
- Smile a little
- Practice mindful breathing
- Observe our in and out-breath
- Breathing in, we know we are breathing in
- Breathing out, we know we are breathing out
- Follow the entire length of our breath
- Be aware of our own presence
- Feel our whole body
- Relax our whole body
- Then, give patient all of our attention
- Look at patient as if he or she is the only person in the world
- Maintain constant eye contact

- Relax our gaze
- Observe his or her facial expression
- Observe his or her body posture and movement
- See patient as a whole person
- Breathe in and out when we find ourselves judging patient
- Breathe in and out when we find ourselves feeling anxious
- Breathe in and out when we find ourselves feeling rushed
- Come back to our breathing gently when we are distracted
- Come back to the present moment
- Come back to our body
- Come back to our presence
- Breathing in, we are completely there for the patient
- Breathing out, we are happy to see the patient
- Be there fully for the patient

Mindful Listening

Introduction

Mindful listening is the second component of MBST. We are all very good at talking. We talk a lot. And we don't allow patient to talk because we think we know a lot but the reality is not. We may be experts in our own field, but patients are experts in their own experiences. Sometimes we are too busy. So we just talk and go, worse than touch and go. We talk and go, leaving patients with a confused look. To understand the experiences of patients, we need to learn to listen.

If patient is talking, we listen. If patient is not talking, we have to know what to ask. Ask using open-ended questions. Can you tell me a little about your experience? Can you tell me more? Is there anything else you want to tell me for me to understand your situation more so I can see how to help? Please share your experience with me. Please let me understand what are your difficulties? Refer to Table 1 for more questions. After asking, we listen attentively. We listen without interrupting. We listen in a way as if the patient is the only person talking to us.

First, we practice mindful breathing as an anchor of our attention. Breathing in, we know we are breathing in. Breathing out, we know we are breathing out. Breathing in a long breath, we know we are breathing in a long breath. Breathing out a long breath, we know we are breathing out a long breath. Breathing in a short breath, we know we are breathing in a short breath. Breathing out a short breath, we know we are breathing out a short breath. Breathing in, we calm and relax our whole body. Breathing out, we smile with love.

Table 1 – Open-ended questions in assessing suffering

Patients
Can you tell me a little about your experience?
How has this illness affected you physically?
What about your emotions?
How have your family been throughout your illness?
What about your friends?
How do you find the doctors and nurses here?
How is it like staying in the hospital?
What things do you believe in that is important to you now?
Is there anything else you would like to share with me?

Family caregivers
Can you tell me a little about your experience taking care of him/her?
How have you been affected physically?
What about your emotions?
How have things changed in the family?
What about your friends?
How have the doctors and nurses been?
How do you find the hospital?
What are the things that are important to you now?
Is there anything else you would like to talk about?

In mindful listening, we listen as we breathe in and out. And we create a safe space for patients to express their experiences and problems. We pay attention to the verbal and non-verbal elements of their speeches in regard to the content, sound, rate, rhythm, pitch and volume. We also pay attention to the silences. We have to be comfortable with these silences. And we continue to pay attention to their facial expression and body language as in the practice of mindful presence.

In the silences, we observe whether they are true silences or whether they are full of psychological 'noises', i.e. our reactions. In mindful listening, once we notice our reactions, we just breathe in and out and let them be as they are without disturbing them. 'Noises' can be cognitive reactions like judgment and automatic thinking; emotional reactions like sadness, anger and boredom; and behavioural reactions like interruption, talking and advicing.

Be mindful of our urge of interruption or talking. Interrupt appropriately with awareness. Try not to interrupt till patients have expressed all they want to express. Sometimes patients will continue to talk after a period of silence. Give patients some time during these silences. Don't interrupt these silences immediately. Give patients time to think or reflect. Give them time to rest in these silences. One more thing, be mindful of our facilitations such as head nodding, filler words, clarification, and paraphrasing. Facilitate appropriately. Don't nod our head excessively, or else it may look like titubation as in cerebellar damage. Nod mindfully.

Listening and care of the dying

Speaking from my own days as a doctor, I failed my post-graduate exams multiple times. I found it particularly difficult to pass my communication station no matter how hard I tried and no matter how many communication classes I attended. It was not until I joined Hospis Malaysia that I found some of the best teachers in communications skills were lurking in palliative care. After a little guidance from my teachers, I passed my exam. I learnt that listening is one of the most essential things in life that I was lacking, and it is never more important than when we are caring for the dying. In care of the dying, deep listening is so important. Listening alone may alleviate some of patients' suffering. And if we listen deep enough, it may even take away their fears of death.

Instructions for mindful listening

- Continue to practice mindful breathing
- Breathing in, we know we are breathing in
- Breathing out, we know we are breathing out
- Breathing in long, we know we are breathing in long
- Breathing out long, we know we are breathing out long
- Breathing in short, we know we are breathing in short
- Breathing out short, we know we are breathing out short
- Be aware of the entire length of our breath
- Be aware of our whole body as we breathe in and out
- Be aware of the rising and falling movement of our body
- Breathe in and out to calm our body down
- Breathe in and out to empty our mind to listen
- Use open-ended questions to ask about patient's experience
- Then, listen to the patient with all of our attention
- Listen to the speech
- Listen to the rate, rhythm, pitch and volume
- Listen to the silences
- Observe how the speech arises from the background of silence
- Observe how the speech disappears into silence
- See whether we can still hear the silences behind the speech
- Listen with an open and curious heart
- Create a safe space for the patient to express
- Listen to what is expressed and what is not expressed
- Listen to understand, not to reply
- What are the feelings of the patient?
- What are the thoughts of the patient?
- Listen to understand what the patient WANTs
- What does the patient want us to know?
- What does the patient want us to say?
- What does the patient want us to do?
- Be mindful of our reactions during listening
- Breathe in and out when we find ourselves judging patient
- Breathe in and out when we feel like interrupting patient

- Breathe in and out when we feel like giving advice prematurely
- Breathe in and out when we notice any countertransferences
- If we are distracted, pay attention to our in and out-breath
- In-out, in-out, in-out
- If we are restless, pay attention to the entire length of breath
- In-in-in, out-out-out
- As we feel less restless, gently increase the gap of silences
- From in-in-in, out-out-out back to in-out, in-out
- In this way, we reduce our inner 'noises'
- We increase our inner 'silences'
- Then we come back to pay complete attention to listening
- And we continue to listen with all of ourselves

Mindful Empathy

Introduction

Empathy means to put ourselves in someone else's shoes to understand his or her thoughts and feelings. This is not to be taken literally because I don't think our feet can fit in everyone else's shoes. If we have heard of Cinderella we will know it is not that easy to fit in someone else's shoes. Her stepsisters tried many attempts but failed. Empathy is an attempt to see from another's perspective. We always cling tightly to our own opinions and ideas but empathy requires us to see from a different angle, from the angle of another person. In doing so, we have to temporarily abandon all our preconceived ideas and judgment.

Through listening mindfully to patients and observing their facial expression, postures and body language, mindful empathy can be practiced to 'enter into' patients to understand their feelings and perspectives. Mindful empathy is practiced first by paying attention to our breathing. Breathing in, we know we are breathing in. Breathing out, we know we are breathing out. After taking a few breaths, we direct our attention to seeing ourselves as patients. We pay attention to their descriptions of experience without any distortion from our own views, opinions or agendas.

We see ourselves going through all those suffering narrated by patients to understand the events that make them suffer; and to understand the actual experiencing of those events. Examples of different types of suffering are included in Table 2. For patients' suffering, it can be broadly divided into two – existential suffering, which means suffering seen from the perspective of events; and experiential suffering, means suffering seen from the perspective of experiences. For caregivers' suffering, it can be divided into three types – suffering that arises from seeing another's suffering, suffering that arises from wanting to relieve another's suffering, and suffering that arises from the action in relieving another's suffering.

Mindful empathy is a practice of objective empathy where we observe the unfolding of subjective empathic experiences objectively in our mind without adding our own ideas, notions, judgments or preconceptions. If we are distracted by our reactions, we let them be as they are without reacting further and gently return our attention to empathy. When we find ourselves overimagining, overgeneralizing or catastrophizing, we come back gently to our breathing, then to empathy.

Practicing mindful empathy, we consciously allow patients to express what they want to express without trying to block any of their expressions. If they are crying, we allow them to cry without asking them to stop crying. If they are angry, we allow them to express their anger without explaining away their anger. If they are worried, we tell them it is ok to worry instead of reassuring them and telling them not to worry. The key practice of empathy is to ALLOW, not blocking. The allowing can be in the form of silence, listening, tuning in, acknowledgment, validation or normalization.

In mindful empathy, we see ourselves going through those loss-related and gain-related events of existential suffering. We observe our feelings and thoughts of experiential suffering. Regarding understanding of feelings and thoughts, the most important thing is to know what patients or family caregivers WANT from us, to know their hopes, wishes, expectations and preferences. In this way, we may be able to know what they want us to say or do.

Table 2 – Types of suffering at the end of life

Patients	
Existential suffering (Suffering seen from the perspective of events)	
<u>Loss-related events</u>	<u>Gain-related events</u>
Loss of function	Diagnosis of a terminal disease
Loss of quality of life	Progression of disease
Loss of hope	Experiencing dying
Dependence on others	Lack of attention from others
Perceived burdening of others	Lack of listening from others
Perceived uselessness	Lack of empathy from others
Witnessing family exhaustion	Mobility restriction in the hospital
Witnessing family grief	Unpalatable hospital food
Experiential suffering (Suffering seen from the perspective of experiences)	
<u>Feelings</u>	<u>Thoughts</u>
Feeling pain and other symptoms	Difficulty in acceptance
Feeling shocked	Choiceless acceptance
Feeling worried	Unfulfilled hope
Feeling scared	Hopelessness
Feeling angry	Hope for sooner death
Feeling bored	Why me?
Feeling lonely	Why now?
Feeling sad	Why do I need to suffer?
Feeling regret	Where is God?
Family caregivers	
Suffering that arises from seeing another's suffering	
Seeing suffering of patient	
Seeing exhaustion of other family members	
Perceived impending death of patient	
Perceived impending absence of patient	

Suffering that arises from wanting to relieve another's suffering
Obsession with giving the best care and ignoring own well-being
Obsession with keeping patient alive at all costs
Compulsion to do something for patient
Feeling helpless and powerless
Suffering that arises from doing something to relieve another's suffering
Experiencing the burden of caring
Having conflict with patient, other family members or healthcare staff
Repercussion on personal and social life

Although mindful presence, mindful listening and mindful empathy are discussed separately in different chapters, they are all linked together in practice. In regard to the *satipatthana*, the practices of mindful presence, mindful listening and mindful empathy help us to UNDERSTAND the feelings, mind and thoughts of another person. With the help of mindful presence and mindful listening, mindful empathy allows us to practice mindfulness of feelings externally (mindfulness of feelings of another person), mindfulness of mind externally (mindfulness of mind of another person) and mindfulness of thoughts externally (mindfulness of thoughts of another person).

In regard to feelings, when patients are feeling happy, we know they are feeling happy; when they are feeling suffering, we know they are feeling suffering; when they are feeling neutral, we know they are feeling neutral. In regard to mind, when patients are having the 'I want'-mind, we know they are having the 'I want'-mind; when they are not having the 'I want'-mind, we know they are not having the 'I want'-mind; when they are having the 'I don't want'-mind, we know they are having the 'I don't want'-mind; when they are not having the 'I don't want'-mind, we know they are not having the 'I don't want'-mind; and when they are having the 'Why me?'-mind, we know they are having the 'Why me?'-mind; when they are not having the 'Why me?'-mind, we know they are not having the 'Why me?'-mind.

Examples of suffering caused by the 'I want' mind include 'I want to be cured', 'I want to be able to do everything myself', 'I want to feel normal back again', 'I want my life back', 'I want my family to feel happy', etc. These mental states cause suffering when what patients want is unfulfilled. On the other hand, examples of suffering caused by the 'I don't want'-mind include 'I don't want to be sick', 'I don't want to feel pain', 'I don't want to suffer', 'I don't want to die', 'I don't want to meet any uncaring doctors and nurses', 'I don't want to stay in the hospital', etc. Patients suffer when they experience what they don't want to experience.

In regard to thoughts, we abide observing the thoughts of patients in terms of the five hindrances. If liking is present in patients, we know 'There is liking in patients'; if liking is not present in patients, we know 'There is no liking in patients'. So are the other four hindrances of disliking, tiredness, agitation and doubt. The main way we can access patients' thoughts is through listening to patients and observing their non-verbal language, not through the superpower of mindreading. Doubt here refers to the hindrance directly related to the practice of mindfulness. It should be absent in patients unless they are aware of mindfulness and they are practicing it. In another lens, doubt can be referred to as unanswered questions that cause suffering, such as why me and where is God.

We abide observing the sense of self in patients. If patients are clinging to their body, we know they are clinging to their body; if patients are clinging to their raw feelings, we know they are clinging to their raw feelings; if patients are clinging to their perceptions, we know they are clinging to their perceptions; if patients are clinging to their thoughts and judgments, we know patients are clinging to their thoughts and judgments; if patients are clinging to their awareness, we know they are clinging to their awareness. Clinging means repetitive thinking and holding on to an object of attention tightly and not willing to stop thinking.

We abide observing thoughts in terms of the six internal and external sense-spheres of patients. When patients express their suffering, we know their suffering is dependent on both the internal and external sense-spheres. We know the sources of their suffering whether it is coming from seeing, hearing, smelling, tasting, feeling or thinking. We know which of the internal and external sense-spheres that trigger their suffering.

The first stage of practicing mindful empathy requires us to see ourselves as patients to understand the presence or absence of the different types of existential and experiential suffering as shown in Table 2. The second stage is to see ourselves as patients to understand the actual psychological processes of suffering. Although each patient experiences suffering differently, the actual psychological processes of suffering follow five common patterns.

First, patients perceive unpleasant events through their six sense-spheres of seeing, hearing, smelling, tasting, feeling and knowing. Second, patients negatively appraise their events as suffering. They appraise through interpreting an event negatively, through comparing themselves with the past and other healthy people, through imagining themselves going through bad things in the future and through believing in a way that is harmful to themselves.

Their cognitive distortions include focusing on the negative, such as unwanted losses and changes, burdening of others, family stress, pain and suffering, poor communication from doctors and nurses and unpleasant stay; ignoring what is good, what they can still do or how they can still live happily despite the disease. They magnify their situation to a greater degree than it is. Sometimes they even catastrophize to the worst possible outcome. They generalize broad assumption by inferring incorrectly from their specific negative experiences. They see their situation in a black-and-white manner, either to recover or die. They feel they 'should' be like this or like that instead of accepting unchangeable things as they are.

Third, patients struggle to accept what is happening to them. They hope things can be different. These are thoughts related to the sense of self, such as 'I want' and 'I don't want'. Patients suffer when they cannot get what they want, and when they experience what they don't want. Fourth, patients experience a wide range of emotions of suffering, such as shock, anger, fear, anxiety, guilt, regret, boredom, loneliness and sadness. Fifth, they perpetuate their suffering through clinging. They pay full attention to their negative perceptions, appraisals, hopes, struggles with acceptance and emotions, and not willing to let go or move forward.

Understanding these five common psychological patterns allows us to have a better idea of what patients are going through so we can think of a way to assist them in relieving their suffering. The reason why suffering remains so prevalent despite the advancement of science and technology is because we have been focusing entirely on modifying the events or external sources of suffering but not on transforming the inner experiences of patients. The 'looking inside' or mindfulness of the body, feelings, mind and thoughts can be the first step to develop insight into patients' suffering. Without a thorough understanding of patients' suffering, we will not be able to assist in alleviating their suffering experiences sufficiently.

Instructions for mindful empathy

- Continue to practice mindful breathing
- Breathing in, we know we are breathing in
- Breathing out, we know we are breathing out
- Breathing in long, we know we are breathing in long
- Breathing out long, we know we are breathing out long
- Breathing in short, we know we are breathing in short
- Breathing out short, we know we are breathing out short
- Be aware of the entire length of our breath
- In-in-in, out-out-out
- In-in-in, out-out-out
- Be aware of our whole body as we breathe in and out
- Be aware of the rising of our chest and abdomen
- Be aware of the falling of our chest and abdomen
- Breathe in and out and let our body calm down naturally
- Slowly, let go of our attachment to our body
- Let go of our feelings
- Let go of our thoughts and opinions
- Let go of our sense of self completely
- See ourselves 'entering into' patient's body
- Experience his or her body
- Experience the body in regard to his or her breathing
- Experience the body in regard to his or her posture
- Experience the body in regard to his or her body movement
- Be aware of the body parts and their nature
- See ourselves feeling patient's feelings
- Experience feelings in regard to the three feeling tones
- Is patient experiencing feeling of *sukha*, *dukkha*, or *upekkha*?
- See ourselves 'entering into' patient's mind
- Experience the mind in regard to the different mental states
- Is his or her mind craving for something pleasant (*raga citta*)?
- Is his or her mind rejecting something unpleasant (*dosa citta*)?
- Is his or her mind confused (*moha citta*)?
- Is his or her mind free from greed, anger and confusion?

- See ourselves thinking patient's thoughts
- Experience thoughts in regard to the five hindrances
- Any liking, disliking, lethargy, restlessness or doubt?
- Experience thoughts in regard to the five aggregates
- Is patient clinging to his or her body?
- Is patient clinging to his or her feelings?
- Is patient clinging to his or her perceptions and appraisals?
- Is patient clinging to his or her hopes, wishes and expectations?
- Is patient clinging to his or her consciousness?
- Experience thoughts in regard to the six sense-spheres
- See the arising of thoughts in patient from seeing
- See the arising of thoughts in patient from hearing
- See the arising of thoughts in patient from smelling
- See the arising of thoughts in patient from tasting
- See the arising of thoughts in patient from feeling
- See the arising of thoughts in patient from thinking
- See ourselves 'entering into' patient's situation
- Be aware of the events that make patient suffer
- Be aware of the actual experiencing of these events
- Observe the arising and the passing away of these experiences
- Perceptions, appraisals, hopes/acceptance, emotions, clinging
- Practice empathy by keeping silence
- Practice empathy by listening with full attention
- Practice empathy by seeing ourselves as patient
- Practice empathy by allowing patient to ventilate feelings
- Practice empathy by acknowledging his or her feelings
- Practice empathy by validating his or her feelings
- Practice empathy by normalizing his or her feelings
- Breathe in and out when we find ourselves overimagining
- Breathe in and out when we feel like blocking any expression
- Breathe in and out when we are affected by vicarious emotions
- Continue to see ourselves as patient
- Continue until we have fully UNDERSTAND patient's situation
- Continue until we know what patient wants us to say or do
- Then, come back to our body and mind
- Come back to our breathing

Books and empathy

I discovered my love of books since I was a pre-schooler. I was so fascinated by the pictures and words in one Giant Dictionary that I carried it wherever I went. The book was really huge compared to my small figure. At the age of four, I volunteered to get enrolled at a kindergarten. It was mostly fun and play. After school, I spent a lot of times at my grandparents' grocery stall reading comics such as Old Master Q and Doraemon. You can say that a big part of my life is mainly about books. If you can't find me in the library, you can probably find me in a bookshop. Working in palliative care, I came to realize that every patient is like a book full of interesting stories. They can be romance, action, adventure, horror, mystery, fantasy or even a mixture of all. If we are kind enough to listen, patients may share their stories with us. So, if patient is a book, then empathy is reading it. If we don't read the pages, we will never know what is inside.

Mindful Compassion

Introduction

In modern society, people are conditioned by social media and commercials to chase materialism. People learn to become more and more materialistic and individualistic. People care a lot more about themselves, not so much about others. It is like survival of the fittest. I don't care about you. I just want to satisfy my own desires. These desires are hot and burning, full of thoughts of wanting more and more. And we are never satisfied with what we have. We just want more, more, more – more money, more fame, more achievement, more praises, more followers in Facebook and Instagram, and more likes. This is why sometimes people say burning desire, like eternal flames; burning ourselves, burning others, consuming everything, causing global warming.

We need less of these desires. We need less except this one desire, i.e. the desire to help, the desire to relieve suffering or COMPASSION. Compassion is a cooling and refreshing emotion. It is free from all burning thoughts. It is cooler than air-conditioning, ice-kacang or Frozen Coke. It cools down other desires. It cools down anger and violence. It cools down pain and suffering. It cools down global warming. It is very refreshing, like sniffing morning fresh air, like sipping Coca-Cola during hot weather, and like splashing ourselves with a bucket of cold water when we are feeling exhausted. We need more compassion, more kindness, more cool. Be compassionate. Be kind. Be cool! Instead of saying 'I don't care', we say 'I care'. We need to practice caring, practice compassion, and practice kindness. Have a little compassion. Have a little kindness. Let us be cool!

So, what is compassion? Some people say compassion is to suffer with. It is like you suffer, I suffer. Is it true? No. If we suffer together with patients, we won't be able to help them. We ourselves probably need some compassion. So, compassion is not to suffer with. Compassion is the perception of another's suffering, coupled with the sincere wish and action to relieve the suffering. Compassion is an indispensable necessity in humanity. Without compassion, the soul of medicine will be lost. We will be 'soulless' doctors. Now, let us first look at the three components of compassion.

The first component of compassion is the perception of another's suffering. We put ourselves in another's shoes to perceive and understand his or her suffering. Without a thorough understanding of what patients are going through and without knowing what patients want us to do to help, we cannot help them. We may even cause more suffering despite our good intention. This is why the first thing about compassion is to completely understand the situations of patients through the practice of mindful empathy.

Once we have understood the situations clearly, once we have understood what patients want us to say or do, we can then proceed to the second component – the intention component. We make a sincere wish for patients to be free from his or her suffering. It is like a prayer. May you be free from your suffering. May you be happy and at ease all the time. We can constantly keep this prayer in our mind as long as patients are still suffering. This prayer is not necessarily directed to one patient only; it can be extended to everyone who is suffering. We can make this sincere wish to do good to others on waking up early in the morning. Then we remind ourselves of this noble thought every now and then throughout the day and just before we sleep.

We can practice compassion meditation 20 minutes every day to increase our compassion. We sit comfortably and relax our body like when we are practicing mindful breathing. We close our eyes. Breathe in and out naturally. Then, we make a wish from the depth of our heart: I am going to dedicate myself in developing compassion for the sake of all beings. Imagine someone we love suffering in front of us. Open our heart to feel the suffering of this person. Feel the suffering from the bottom of our heart. Rest in this suffering for a few moments. Make a sincere wish for this person to be free from suffering: may he or she be free from all suffering. Imagine directing our compassion toward this person. Rest in this compassion for the next few moments. Now, imagine extending compassion to all family members, friends, strangers, enemies and all beings. Take time to deepen our compassion to each group. At the end, see the whole universe filled with boundless compassion.

Third, the action component, if we just make a wish and stop there, nothing will happen. We have to take action to fulfil our wish. Without this third component, compassion is just empty vessel making noise only. To make compassion complete, we need to find out how to help patients after thoroughly understanding their situations. We need to speak and act in such a way that can palliate the suffering of patients.

Since there are infinite types of suffering, we have to find INFINITE ways to reduce suffering. If patients are in pain, we find ways to reduce their pain. If patients feel cold, we find them a blanket. If patients want to drink, we help them to get their cups. If patients want to cry, we allow them to cry. If patients want to go home, we help them to go home. There are in fact infinite ways to reduce suffering, but all of them originated from a single source, i.e. COMPASSION.

Compassion is not rocket science. Yes, we need to be fully equipped with medical knowledge and skills to alleviate patients' suffering, but at times, small act of kindness alone will do. Once I had a patient dying in ICU, what her family wanted from us was to just keep her in ICU instead of transferring her out to the general ward. We spoke to the ICU team and they agreed to keep the patient there until she died. And she died after a couple of hours. There are infinite ways to relieve suffering, but what this family needed was just one simple way.

Compassion is one of the four practices of kindness – namely love, compassion, joy and equanimity. These four practices are interlinked. They are called the Four Immeasurables (*Appamana Cetovimutti* in Pali) because they can dissolve the boundaries that constrain us. They open our heart in limitless ways so we can embrace countless people. According to the Four Immeasurables, immeasurable love (*metta*) means to bring happiness to countless people; immeasurable compassion (*karuna*) means to alleviate suffering of countless people; immeasurable joy (*mudita*) means to rejoice at the happiness of countless people; and immeasurable equanimity (*upekkha*) means to let go of our sense of self to help countless others in a selfless manner.

Before we can reach the level of immeasurable compassion, we need to first practice mindful compassion. Without being mindful, compassion can be fatiguable. Many people experience compassion fatigue when they are trying to help patients. Many people suffer together with patients, or are overwhelmed by suffering. We call this compassion suffering. Compassion has many challenges. When we perceive another's suffering, we can experience vicarious traumatization or anticipatory grief. When we intend to relieve the suffering of another, we may feel helpless and powerless, or we may be troubled by obsessive thoughts in giving the best care. When we act to relieve suffering, we may experience resistance from patients, family members or other healthcare providers. Sometimes we neglect our own well-being. That is why compassion without mindfulness can cause suffering.

In practicing mindful compassion, first we pay attention to our breath. Breathing in, we know we are breathing in. Breathing out, we know we are breathing out. We pay attention to the entire length of our breath. In-in-in; out-out-out. In-in-in; out-out-out. We feel our whole body as we breathe in and out and we relax our whole body. Then we consciously cultivate the intention to relieve patient's suffering. We repeat phrases such as 'May you be free from suffering' or 'May you be happy and at ease', silently in our mind. Likewise, we can memorize and repeat the Indian sage Shantideva's aspiration: For as long as space endures, and as long as human beings exist, until then may I too remain to dispel the miseries of the world. After that, we pay attention to the thoughts and feelings of compassion that arise. And we let these thoughts and feelings manifest in our speech and actions.

Being mindful of what patients want us to say and do from the practice of empathy, we speak and act mindfully in consistent with the hopes, wishes and expectations of patients. We speak and act with clear comprehension (sampajanna). We are clearly aware of the purpose of our speech and action. Are we doing good with our speech and action? Or are we doing harm? Is our speech or action appropriate? Is it the right time, place or person? Which foundations of mindfulness are we practicing? We are clearly aware. We are also clearly aware of the reality. We know the changing nature of our speech and action (temporal reality); we know the conditioned nature of our speech and action (spatial reality); and we know the unsatisfactory nature of our speech and action (psychological reality – that we cannot satisfy everyone).

When we speak, we know we are speaking. When we are speaking fast, we know we are speaking fast. When we are speaking slowly, we know we are speaking slowly. We speak in a manner to calm down patients' suffering. As we speak, we can continue to pay attention to our breathing. And then we may notice that speaking occurs during our breathing out. We can pay attention to the movement of our mouth, tongue and throat during speaking.

The next thing is we make use of our rate, rhythm, volume, pitch, intonation and silences to relieve suffering. We make use of our eye contact, facial expression and body language to convey our care. We are mindful of the content of our speech in such a way that at the very least we do not do harm with it. At best we make full use of the speech content, paralanguage and body language to relieve suffering of patients, and to bring happiness to them.

Apart from mindful speaking, we also pay attention to every act that we do. When we smile, we act clearly knowing. When we lift a blanket to cover patient, we act clearly knowing. When we adjust the slippers of patient, we act clearly knowing. When we pass patient his or her glasses, we act clearly knowing. When we perform mouth care, we act clearly knowing. When we give medicine, we act clearly knowing.

In this way, when we perform any activity, we perform with clear comprehension of the purpose and proportionality of the activity, the appropriateness, the field of practice and the reality – temporal, spatial and psychological. We recognize the arising and fading away of our experiences. Recognizing to the extent just enough to be clearly aware of the activity from time to time; abiding independently not clinging to anything in the world.

The practice of mindful compassion builds on the previous components of MBST. It cannot be separated from them. Mindful presence and mindful listening are all-important parts of mindful empathy. Mindful empathy constitutes the perception component of mindful compassion. Then, mindful compassion continues with compassionate wishing – the intention component, followed by mindful speaking and mindfulness of activities in relieving suffering – the action component. Therefore, the core ingredient in MBST is the mindful compassion component.

Mindful compassion is a process-orientated compassion. It focuses on the process of compassion rather than the goal. Common reactions that can arise during the practice of mindful compassion include negative judgments, being overly-obsessed with care, having excessive concerns in fixing the suffering and excessive attachment to the goal of relieving suffering. Whenever we are distracted by any of these reactions, we breathe in and out and gently bring our attention back to compassion. And repeat our magic phrases, 'May you be free from suffering', 'May you be happy and at ease'.

Instructions for mindful compassion

- Continue mindful breathing
- Breathing in, we know we are breathing in
- Breathing out, we know we are breathing out
- Breathing in long, we know we are breathing in long
- Breathing out long, we know we are breathing out long
- Breathing in short, we know we are breathing in short
- Breathing out short, we know we are breathing out short
- Be aware of the entire length of our breath
- Be aware of our whole body as we breathe in and out
- Be aware of the rising and falling movement of our body
- Breathe in and out to calm our body down

- Then, cultivate compassion consciously
- Start with perception of patient's suffering
- Open our heart to feel patient's suffering
- Feel his or her suffering from the bottom of our heart
- Rest in this feeling of suffering for a few moments
- Breathe in and breathe out while feeling the suffering
- Then, continue with the intention to relieve patient's suffering
- Make a sincere wish for patient to be free from all suffering
- "May you be free from all suffering"
- "May you be happy and at ease"
- Imagine directing our compassion toward the patient
- Rest in this feeling of compassion for a few moments
- Breathe in and breathe out while feeling the compassion
- Then, continue with the action component when time is right
- Speak with clear comprehension to comfort patient
- Act with clear comprehension to alleviate patient's suffering
- Continue to anchor our attention with our breathing
- Once we feel we are distracted, gently come back to our breath
- Let go of our judgment of patient
- Let go of our excessive obsession with care
- Let go of our excessive concern in fixing suffering
- Let go of our excessive attachment to our goals
- Breathe when we are emotionally affected by patient
- Breathe when we feel guilty of not doing enough
- Breathe when we feel helpless not knowing what to do
- Breathe when we feel like saying something unnecessarily
- Breathe when we feel like doing something unnecessarily
- Breathe when we feel like avoiding patient we don't like
- Continue to pay attention to our breathing
- Continue to express compassion in our speech and action

Bringing peace out of the monastery

If you want me to describe my experience staying in the Abode of Still Thoughts back in 1998 at Hualien, Taiwan, I will use three words: clean, quiet and peaceful. The monastery was very clean. It reminded me about my OCD-ness during school days. The monks and nuns spent a lot of time in cleaning. Besides, every task was performed with full attention. So, the monastery was wrapped in complete silence. When we walked, we walked in a line quietly. When we ate, we ate without talking. Whatever food we took, we finished it. After finishing, we poured water into our bowl and drank all the remnants so that we were not wasting any food. Silence was very palpable. The only things that broke the silence in the monastery were sounds from nature and voices from chanting. It was such a peaceful experience. The silence was not only outside but also inside. My mind was very quiet too.

After coming back to Malaysia, the challenge to me is how to bring that sense of peace into my ordinary life. I can enjoy all the peace by myself in a monastery, but the peace becomes meaningful only if I can bring it out of the monastery into my daily life or share it with others. Then, I discovered a simple way. Instead of listening to music while I drive to work every morning, I listen to a guided meditation CD on peace by Tulku Thondop Rinpoche. I continue to practice mindful breathing while I listen to the CD. And that gives me a similar sense of peace like when I was staying in the monastery, but this time in the middle of the morning traffic jam. Sometimes I can still feel the peace when I see patients in the ward. And I believe that sense of peace may help to calm some patients down in the midst of their grief.

Mindfulness of Boundaries

Introduction

Before we talk about boundaries, let us revise the *Satipatthana Sutta* a little. *Satipatthana Sutta*: In regard to the body [feelings, mind and thoughts], one abides observing the body [etc.] internally, or one abides observing the body [etc.] externally, or one abides observing the body [etc.] **BOTH INTERNALLY AND EXTERNALLY**. One abides observing the nature of arising in the body [etc.], the nature of disappearing and both. Mindfulness that 'there is a body' [etc.] is established to the extent necessary for bare knowledge and continuous mindfulness. And one abides independently, not clinging to anything in the world.

This last chapter is about observing the body, feelings, mind and thoughts **BOTH INTERNALLY AND EXTERNALLY**. It is about practicing mindfulness of self and others together. Although we cannot observe an object both internally and externally simultaneously, we can alternate between the two modes. We maintain awareness of the boundary between self and others. We maintain awareness of our body, feelings, mind and thoughts and patient's body, feelings, mind and thoughts.

Boundary has been described as the mutually understood, unspoken, physical and emotional limits of the relationship between the trusting patient and the caring physician or provider. Examples of potential boundary issues comprise receiving gifts from patients, giving out phone number to patients, socializing with patients outside of the clinical setting and revealing excessive personal information to patients.

Definite boundary issues include accepting money from a patient or family member, attending to patient to fulfil a personal need, attempting a deathbed conversion, giving in to request for futile treatment and giving in to request for hastening of death. Although sometimes crossing boundaries can enhance patient care, boundary awareness is essential to avoid boundary issues that are harmful to the therapeutic relationship and boundary violation.

Mindfulness of boundaries is paying attention to personal and professional boundaries. Once we have grounded ourselves by practicing mindful breathing, we direct our conscious attention to boundary issues that arise during our practices of presence, listening, empathy and compassion. We consciously monitor our physical and emotional limits of the relationship between patients and us. We consciously maintain our awareness when boundaries are approached. After careful reflection, we cross boundaries consciously only if we are convinced that crossing boundary in a particular situation is beneficial to patient and the therapeutic relationship, without violating professional conduct.

Mindfulness of boundaries is a practice of self-awareness. It is a practice of simultaneously attending to the care of patients and the care of ourselves. Compassion is incomplete if it is just one-way compassion. Compassion should be a two-way process – compassion for others and compassion for ourselves. If we notice ourselves neglecting our own well-being while caring for others, we breathe in and out and try to remember to take care of ourselves. If we notice ourselves reacting negatively to a situation, we breathe in and out and try to return our attention back to monitoring our personal and professional limits. If we notice ourselves crossing boundary that can harm patient or ourselves, we breathe in and out and abandon our intention.

Instructions for mindfulness of boundaries

- Continue mindful breathing
- Breathing in, we know we are breathing in

- Breathing out, we know we are breathing out
- In-out, in-out, in-out
- Then, observe both breathing of ourselves and patient's
- In-out (own), in-out (own), in-out (own)
- In-out (patient), in-out (patient), in-out (patient)
- Breathing in long, we know we are breathing in long
- Breathing out long, we know we are breathing out long
- Breathing in short, we know we are breathing in short
- Breathing out short, we know we are breathing out short
- Be aware of the entire length of our breath
- In-in-in, out-out-out
- Then, observe the entire length of both our breath and patient's
- In-in-in (own), out-out-out (own)
- In-in-in (patient), out-out-out (patient)
- Be aware of our whole body as we breathe in and out
- Then, pay attention to both our own body and patient's
- Observe both our own body postures and patient's
- Observe both our own physical activities and patient's
- Contemplate both our own physical constituents and patient's
- Contemplate the nature of decay of both our body and patient's
- Observe both our own feelings and patient's
- Observe both our own mental states and patient's
- Observe both our own thoughts and patient's
- Be aware of our personal boundary
- Notice the boundary between self and others
- Notice our own judgment versus patient's thoughts
- Notice our own emotions versus patient's emotions
- Be aware of self-care versus patient care
- Be aware of time constraint versus presence
- Be aware of countertransferences versus listening
- Be aware of vicarious traumatization versus empathy
- Be aware of compassion fatigue versus compassion
- Be aware of our professional boundary too
- Cross boundary consciously only if we are convinced that crossing boundary in that particular situation is beneficial

to patient and the therapeutic relationship without violating our professional conduct or compromising equity of care
- Come back to our breath gently when
- We are judging patient for making unreasonable request
- We are judging ourselves for not fulfilling the request
- We are feeling guilty
- We are feeling helpless
- We feel like crossing boundary that can harm patient
- We feel like avoiding patient due to boundary issues
- Maintain self-awareness throughout the encounter

Going home and mindfulness

Home is more than just a place where one lives. It is a place where the heart is. That's why people say, "there is no place like home". Going home is like going back to our source, our origin, our root. Every time when we go home, we feel very peaceful and relaxed. We don't feel like doing anything. We just be, like having the most chilled holiday, lying on a beach, feeling the breeze and drinking a coconut. In the same sense, mindfulness is a ticket to go home. It is a ticket to a place where our heart is. It can bring us to a place beyond the limits of our mind. That place is our source, our origin, our root. When we arrive, we feel completely peaceful and truly relaxed. We don't have to do anything. We just be, resting in the nature of our mind, like having a psychological holiday, seeing things as they are, free from conceptualization, judgment, duality. This is how we should practice mindfulness, GO HOME!

Printed in the United States
By Bookmasters